Kareen Zebroff, happily married mother of three, bestselling author of four books, lecturer-demonstrator, researcher, Yoga and Nutrition expert, organic gardener and health food cook, qualified school teacher, sparkles with good health and *joie de vivre*. For the seven short years since she first took up Yoga she has changed from tense and brittle to graceful and flexible. Good nutrition practices and the soothing Yoga poses have transformed an overweight housewife with the debilitating symptoms of anxiety, irritability and lack of energy, into a relaxed and joyous person. Now she shares her secret with you . . .

ALSO by KAREEN ZEBROFF

THE ABC OF YOGA
YOGA AND NUTRITION

and published by CORGI BOOKS

Beauty Through Yoga

Kareen Zebroff

CORGI BOOKS
A DIVISION OF TRANSWORLD PUBLISHERS LTD

BEAUTY THROUGH YOGA

A CORGI BOOK 0 552 98059 5

First publication in Great Britain

PRINTING HISTORY

Corgi edition published 1978

Illustrations by Bee Walters
Weightloss diet research by Natalie Rogers, B.P.H.E.
Photographs by Duncan McDougall, F.R.P.S.

Corgi Books are published by Transworld Publishers Ltd.,
Century House, 61–63 Uxbridge Road, Ealing, London, W5 5SA

Made and printed in Great Britain by
Richard Clay (The Chaucer Press), Ltd., Bungay, Suffolk.

PREFACE

Dear Readers:

This is a highly personal book. In a way, I wrote it just as much for myself as for you. My principal reason was to make the many aspects of Yoga work for us in our everyday life: to westernize it, to make it applicable to modern living. The western mind is impatient, it likes quick results, it is a world of ACTION. For such a world, Karma Yoga — the Yoga of Action — is ideal.

In this book we make a new beginning. Man is nothing if he does not constantly strive for perfection, for improvement. But since this is an "instant" age, I wrote the book for fourteen days only. That brings it within the grasp of everyone. The reformed Alcoholic pledges *not* to drink one day at a time, because he knows he has the discipline for that only. The thought of a year's, even a week's, dryness would defeat him. That is why our "rejuvenation" program is also short. Fourteen days of discipline is entirely bearable, when you know that all of you benefits — mentally and physically.

For, you are a whole person with a body and a mind, an exterior and an interior. These entities are indivisible, interdependent. Therefore any self-improvement program must deal with the four separate aspects which, together, form a total unit: your body, your nutrition, your outer image, your mind. An exercise book for only your muscles ignores the organic man; a book on nutrition is treating only half the body; a book on beauty is useless if it does not consider nutrition; a book on meditation will never be fully effective if an unfit body distracts the mind. That is why I combined four subjects in one book. It harnesses four weak units into one strong, healthy POWER.

In this book, I am not going to ask you to exercise for an hour, or half-an-hour or even 10 minutes. All I want you to promise yourself is a beauty-exercising program of 5 minutes. This way you won't be able to say that you don't have the time. I know perfectly well that once you have gotten down on the floor and have experienced the delightful stretching exercises of Yoga, you will get charmed into a *longer* work-out time. Exercising (Yoga or otherwise) is a discipline which needs daily repetition, however short, to be fully effective. And if you combine these five minutes with the use of what I call TRIGGER-YOGA, you are practising Yoga all day long. Make a habit of letting your mind trigger the thought 'Yoga' every time an habitual or repetitive situation occurs: i.e., pull your tummy in every time you bend over, balance on one leg while you are on the phone, stick out your tongue in the *Lion* every time you come to a red light in the car, do an intense forward bend every time you brush your hair. In other words, let Yoga and exercise become a part of your whole daily routine.

Although I have devised a Yoga program for 14 days, it is entirely possible to repeat each or any of the sections, separately of the others, for reinforcement of what you have learned. However, keep the Total Concept in mind. Regard these two weeks not as an isolated incident, but as a positive step towards an improved life style.

K. H. Z.

Vancouver, B.C.
September, 1975

TABLE OF CONTENTS
FOURTEEN DAY REJUVENATION PROGRAM

Page

Symbols used throughout the book

Image Section

Hatha Yoga Section

Nutrition and Diet Section

Meditation Section

INTRODUCTION

What is Beauty?

The ideal 'beauty' is one who is true to herself. She knows herself and has accepted herself as she is. The clever French woman always looks chic because she realistically analyzes her body and dresses accordingly for the rest of her life: with a basic dress-pattern which hides the flaws and brings out the good points of her personal proportions. To me, beauty is proportion. My doctor father always felt that men's legs were more beautiful than women's. I believe that to be true if you speak in general terms. In a group of 50 men and 50 women, more men will have attractive legs than women, because the men have fewer flabby thighs, less varicose veins, swollen ankles or fat knees than their female counterparts. All these ailments disturb the essential 'golden measure' that may have existed at a younger age. This measure has more to do with mathematical equations than with weight. For instance, it is entirely possible for an Amazon to be beautiful, since her ample bosom is balanced by her generous hips, her sturdy legs by her feisty arms. A woman, then, need not be model-thin to be attractive. What she must bear in mind is: "Is my weight distribution proportionate? AM I TRIM?"

Medical men divide us into three distinct body types: the tall, slender body, the athletically sturdy body and the roly-poly type. Within each group you will find many variations or extremes but you also encounter true beauty no matter what the basic body build may be. This brings us back to proportion.

The ideal beauty does not belong to one of the three body type groups. She is the one who carries herself with poise and grace, who looks vibrantly healthy, neither starved nor over-indulged. Within the structure of body-types you again find sub-structures of big — medium — and small-boned. It is this, in particular, which explains the puzzling phenomenon of the two girls of similar height and weight — one of whom looks just right and the other overweight. The reason may be physical condition-ing. This means that you can look voluptuously "stacked" because you are trim. As soon as the muscle turns to fat, however, the silhouette thickens and softens, the proportion of the curves melts away.

This is the place to impress upon women the importance of being realistic in their goal, and of dismissing once and for all the false notion of food intake being the chief villain in a flabby figure. The true problem is one of deficiency — deficiency of EXERCISE. In a recent study by the Canadian government it was found that overweight people do not necessarily eat more, they simply exercise less!

Beauty is a matter of taste and, happily, tastes vary. You must accept from the very beginning that you are basically BEAUTIFUL! After all, true beauty shines forth from within. It is more than a feature, it is an attitude. Charm, warmth, serenity, interest in other people, a sense of humour, graceful movement, cleanliness and an attractively firm body all add up to true feminine beauty all over the world.

If you need improvement, dieting will only result in general weight loss, not in spot-reducing or fitness. Stand naked in front of a mirror and take stock. First, how's the proportion? Second, what needs to be shaped? Third, what has to be pulled in, tightened? Be honest. Be realistic in your goal. Accept your individual beauty potential. Be the trimmest, not the thinnest weight for YOU. By all means keep your natural curves. Only a very high cheekboned, small-boned woman can afford to look thin. The rest of us can look years younger than our age simply by looking healthy and natural, not desperate. Personality plays a large part in all but a two-dimensional photo. A tired, tense woman, dully dragging her overweight body like a burden, is ugly no matter what her facial features may be. It becomes necessary in any exercising program, then, to work on one's mental outlook along with the body's improvement. One of the most powerful pieces of advice ever given to me was to 'cultivate a quality of joy'.

Enthusiasm is another positive feeling which will not tolerate a wrinkled brow, a hang-dog expression or a tense-lipped look. You have heard of the technique of making yourself feel better by 'whistling a happy tune to give you courage when you're afraid.' The same principle applies to a look of beauty. No matter what shape you are in, straightening your shoulders, putting a happy look on your face and thinking positive thoughts has a beautifying effect.

What Kareen's Nutritious Weight Loss Diet is all About

This diet was designed by me for YOU. Using five years of experience in the nutrition field, where I interviewed some of America's greatest nutrition experts on T.V., I considered a diet that is not just quick weight loss at a terrible cost to the body. Instead my diet is unique in that my nutrition advisers and I sat down and carefully designed, weighed and researched a balanced, safe and NUTRITIOUS weightloss-diet for you. It is totally self-sufficient in itself, but we have given you the choice of, and guidance with, extra supplements, if you wish to take them. It is my suggestion that you make yourself familiar with our vitamin and mineral charts and check for deficiency symptoms now and then — not just as you go through the diet, but all year-round. The first supplements to consider are:

1 Halibut or cod liver oil capsule (10,000 A, 400 D) daily.
A good Vitamin B Compound tablet once daily.
1 Magnesium oxide tablet between lunch and dinner.
200 units of Vitamin E — 1 tablet daily.
6 dessicated liver tablets — 2 after every meal daily.

Remember that these are just what their names imply: supplements to the daily diet, not food in themselves. We do not prescribe them, we only offer you the information on them. And, instead of giving you the nutrition information all in one huge meal, so-to-speak, we have separated it into palatable little "snacks" spread out over the 14 days of the diet. This allows you food for thought as well as for the stomach.

Our diet is unique. It works well because it . . .

a. promotes a feeling of well-being and energy (no irritability, feeling chilly, or weakness);

b. provides the necessary nutrients for good health as you lose weight: vitamins, minerals, proteins and fatty acids;

c. keeps the blood sugar from dipping by the timing and the contents of the meals — you avoid the hypoglycemia cycle of high and low spirits and energy;

d. allows for psychological satisfaction (on a diet you need all the help you can get) by a built-in system of rewards to keep you going: bananas, apricots, almonds, honey, peanut butter;

e. takes in consideration *food combining* so that your digestion is smoothly efficient — no gassiness;

3

f. consists of only 1050 calories, so cleverly distributed over 6 satisfying meals that you never feel hungry. It is a fact that a person on a 1000 calorie diet which includes 6 meals loses more weight than one on a three meal diet;

g. considers even trace-nutrients. For instance, we included food rich in phosphorus to keep you from getting jumpy. We deliberately planned for potassium (cantaloupe) to help rid the body of waste products such as water;

h. can be combined with the new and very successful diet by Mary Ann Cranshaw which says: On any *1000* calorie diet add:
   1 tbsp. lecithin
   6 kelp tablets after every meal
   1 tsp. apple cider vinegar with the kelp tablets
   50 mg. vitamin B-6

i. can be repeated as often as you like if you add Vit. C, calcium tablets and kelp tablets (for iodine) the next time around. If you repeat, intersperse a week or two of *normal* eating (be careful, the temptation is to overeat). Recent studies with rats have shown that a diet cycle of three repetitions, with time off between, stabilizes the weight.

j. gives alternatives if you have a particular food dislike. But please stick to our suggestions; they are carefully planned;

k. allows you to switch days (i.e. Day 7 for Day 3) though not the individual meal within the days (i.e. do *not* transfer Day 3 lunch for Day 7 lunch). This is nice if you absolutely loathe liver or fish, for instance. However, the liver was carefully planned for nutrient content and if you substitute for liver days, please take extra dessicated liver tablets.

l. will permit you to leave out Day 1, if you are totally turned off by the thought of fasting.

m.provides nutrition-laden calories. When you go out and buy the ingredients, please remember that you are not wasting your money on empty calories (see "What calories are" on page 54) but that every penny buys good food loaded with vitamins, minerals, linoleic acid and proteins which keep you and your family healthy.

How to Prepare for your Diet

Before you start this diet get yourself a little notebook to record exactly: what you eat all day long; when you have the greatest urge to eat; what satisfied you the most today; how you ate and so on. For the first entry write down what you ate the day before the diet. Start with breakfast and include every bite until you went to bed. Be honest. Then tomorrow follow the diet described below and note any deviations in your notebook.

Weigh yourself on Day 1 and again on Day 7 and Day 14, always at the same time of day. Weighing yourself every day is not wise because weight loss is not evident every day.

Prepare the necessary ingredients for the interesting menus laid out for you. After you have followed this regime, you will undoubtedly feel the value of maintaining some of these foods in your normal eating habits.

This suggested shopping list is provided for your convenience:

liquid unpasteurized honey, molasses, flaked nutritional yeast, raw wheat germ, safflower oil (cold pressed, non-hydrogenated), non-homogenized peanut butter (no salt, no additives), hulled sunflower seeds, dried apricots, non-instant skim milk powder or soy flour, apple cider vinegar, herb teas, alfalfa sprouts or water cress, vanilla soy protein powder, almonds (unsalted, skins on), vegetable salt.

No sugar or condiments, mustard, ketchup is allowed. All meals on the diet are to be flavoured with a vegetable salt or mineral salt *only*.

Very Important: No meals should be *missed*. The diet is designed to keep blood sugar from dipping too low. No extra snacks are allowed. But in-between treats have been carefully planned to satisfy your appetite and your hunger and to keep your energy level high.

When we designed it we thought of your total health, not just your fat cells.

Please check with your doctor if it is safe for you to diet for medical considerations.

Day 1

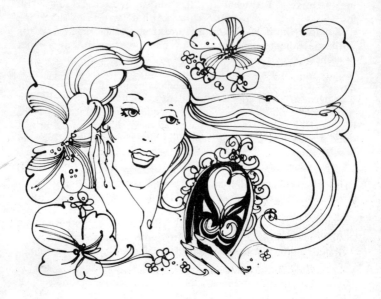

FACE – SKIN

What You Should Know!

— The skin is the largest organ in your body. Its functions are: to regulate body temperature, to synthesize Vitamin D from sunshine, and to eliminate wastes by sweating and by constantly sloughing off cells.

— The beauty of the skin is in direct proportion to moisture content, to positive thinking, to exercise, and, most important of all, to the nutritive elements brought to it through the bloodstream.

— Your skin is considered OILY if it is shiny again within one hour after washing. Test by pressing a facial tissue against the skin, hold it up to the light and see if it shows telltale signs of transparent areas of oil. Oily skin is usually large-pored, coarse, sallow-looking, and has blackheads and open pores. Don't despair. Oily skin looks young longer than the other types.

- Your skin is NORMAL if it is hardly any bother, doesn't peel or flake and has no pimples.
- Your skin is DRY if it is fine-pored, pinky-looking and feels taut within an hour after washing.
- Only a few of the 55 muscles of the face move the mouth and eye area, most of the others are concerned solely with your expression, particularly where several of them are attached to the skin and form a dimple or potential folds and lines.
- An unmarked older face probably mirrors a shallow person.
- A happy, expressive face exercises its muscles constantly, thereby toning the skin.
- Exposing the face to the mid-day sun or prolonged sunbathing exhausts the skin's healing ability.
- Smoking wrinkles and dries the skin.
- Rapid weight losses cause sagging and collapsing of the muscles.
- Stretching the skin through inexpert massaging or too enthusiastic cleansing does irreparable damage.
- In the winter months, central heating and overheated cars dry the skin.

What You Can Do!

1. Unsaturated fatty acids such as LECITHIN and cold-pressed unhydrogenated plant oils are necessary for smoothness from the inside-out.

2. Proteins are used for cell-repair and firm muscles.

3. Vitamin A supplies food to the layer of fat just beneath the skin. In the face, this fat is a prerequisite for every woman's beauty.

4. Vitamin B-2 and B-6, always taken with a B-complex tablet or 1 - 3 tbsp. of flaked brewer's yeast, are excellent for the skin.

5. Vitamin C prevents broken capillaries.

6. Iodine (in kelp or iodized table salt), and iron make for a rosy complexion.

7. Vitamin E regenerates the skin cells and gives a soft look.

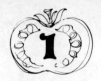

Notes to Dieter

1. Isn't it a nice surprise to find dried apricots, almonds and sunflower seeds in our diet? The fruit sugar in the apricots raises the blood sugar naturally and quickly while the nuts continue to keep the energy level up, through their oil and protein content, for several hours. These seeds are a good source of minerals, vitamins, oil, protein and thereby energy. Apricots and their seeds may be one of the reasons that the people of the famed Hunza tribe live so long.

2. To keep you from feeling hungry and chilled — as often happens with the usual diet — we were careful to include a sufficient daily allowance of fatty acids in our menus. The protein and oil in peanut butter, for example, take considerably longer to pass through the stomach than do carbohydrates. The result: a feeling of satisfaction for up to five hours. Sweets and other carbohydrates, however, have you feeling hungry again as soon as one hour after eating. The salad oils, nuts and butter in our diet also help to avoid the gaunt and wrinkled look that often accompanies dieting. Oil is needed as well for controlling water retention (2 tbsp. of unhydrogenated, cold-pressed oil a day can help to lose many watery pounds). Of interest for the reluctant dieter: if essential fatty acids are missing from the diet, sugar turns to fat more quickly.

3. We need bread. It is one of the reasons our forefathers had the energy to expend great physical effort in their hard daily lives, and that heart attacks were considerably fewer. A slice of *wholewheat bread* is a natural source of good, balanced health (see our after-the-diet recipes in back). So-called "enriched" foods are laughable. Over 20 nutrients may have been removed through the process of refining, and only 5 or so are put back — often synthetic.

4. You'll be delighted to find potatoes on the menu. This is another misunderstood food which, however, was invaluable in such famine-stricken areas as Ireland and Europe after the wars. A medium-sized potato actually has less caloric content than 1/2 cup of cottage-cheese; however, it must be cooked right, always in its jacket. This is a much-maligned vegetable which is really an excellent source of Vitamin C, potassium and some protein.

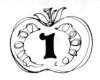

5. All weight-conscious readers should perk up when they hear that by the simple act of adding iron to their diet, as we do in ours, they can drop pounds. There is no excuse for an iron deficiency — molasses, liver and wheat germ are excellent sources and, if necessary, iron tablets are readily available. (See Anemia, Day 14).

KAREEN'S NUTRITIOUS WEIGHT LOSS DIET

More Notes to Dieter

Our first dieting day is the hardest, but it is designed to rid the body of toxins. The detoxifying drink is taken at least five times during the day or as many times as you have the urge to eat. By using the lemon and molasses you are giving your body a feed of vitamins and minerals as it gets a thorough cleansing.

Detoxifying Drink

MIX: 2 tbsp. lemon juice
1 tbsp. molasses, or less, to taste
1 - 8 oz. glass of warm water.

Please rinse your mouth carefully after each glass — lemon and molasses should not stay in contact with the teeth for long. Do not fast on a day where you have lots of physical activity or mental stress.

At the end of 24 hours of a detoxifying diet, the first meal is designed to be easy on your digestive system. You are given enough to eat, but very little protein is included. The emphasis is on fruit and vegetables for better elimination through bulk. In case you get hungry, make yourself a drink of herbal tea; other than water, you should only drink what is permitted on the diet and nothing else.

Our breakfasts are planned to give a substantial beginning to every day, to build up and maintain the blood sugar level for energy all day long. The choice of cantaloupe for fruit is deliberate for its unusually high potassium content. Potassium regulates the water retention in the tissues and corrects any imbalance of sodium in the body.

9

HEAD AND FACE

Breathing exercise for today is the **Beauty Breath**.

1. Sit comfortably in any cross-legged position.
2. Raise arms inhaling deeply.
3. Bend forward from the waist retaining the breath.
4. Hold for 5 seconds.
5. Exhale while straightening.
6. Lower arms and relax.
7. Repeat 4 to 5 times.

Forward Bend Standing — a nice warmup because it improves circulation to the head, working on the wrinkles and complexion while giving a feeling of alertness.

Technique:

1. Stand, with the feet slightly apart.
2. Inhale, raise your hands slowly above your head. (Figure 1)
3. Exhale, bend forward slowly from the waist in a curling motion, dropping your head first and then unfurling each vertebra until you can go no further.
4. Keeping your arms beside your ears, let your body hang forward by its own weight for a few seconds. (Figure 2)
5. Grasp your ankles, or whatever you can comfortably reach, and dig your chin into the neck.
6. Bend your elbows to the side and give a gentle downward and inward stretch, attempting to get your head as close to the knees as possible. (Figure 3)
7. Hold for 5 - 30 seconds, breathing normally.
8. Inhale. Straighten up very slowly, keeping the arms beside the ears and curling the spine up.
9. Repeat twice more.

Do's and Don'ts:

DO NOT bounce or jerk in order to bring your head closer to your knees.

DO NOT worry how far your hands are from the floor, rather how far your head is from your knees.

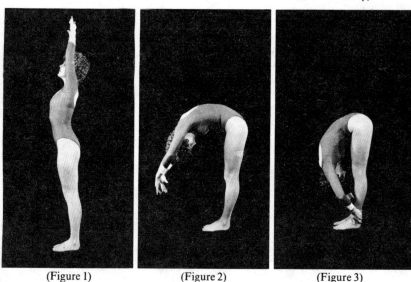

| (Figure 1) | (Figure 2) | (Figure 3) |

The Lion — reduces the tension in the whole facial area, smoothing lines and wrinkles as it tightens and firms the muscles of the face, neck and throat.

Technique:

1. Sit in a kneeling position, toes tucked under and place the hands on the thighs, palms down. (Figure 4)
2. Spread the fingers and slide them forward until the tips touch the floor.
3. Bend your body forward, buttocks off the heels, arms straight. (Figure 5)
4. Open your eyes as wide as possible.
5. Stick your tongue out as far as it will go, attempting to touch the tip of your chin. (Figure 6)
6. Hold 15 seconds.
7. Sit back, pull in your tongue and relax completely.
8. Repeat twice more.

Do's and Don'ts:

DO stick your tongue out completely for a good stretch.
DO NOT be surprised if you have a gagging sensation for a while.
DO the Lion at the sun with the eyes closed.
DO enjoy the marvellous feeling of tension draining away when
    you sit back.

(Figure 4)

(Figure 5)

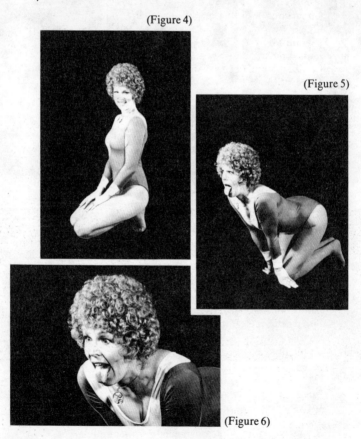

(Figure 6)

Smile-up — tightens all the muscles from your chest to your forehead.

Technique:

1. Put some oil or cream around your eyes to avoid creasing.
2. Press the heels of your palms on the corners of your eyes to prevent crows' feet from forming. (Figure 7)
3. Open your mouth slightly, about 3 cm. (1") and smile up, lifting the upper lip and cheek muscles at the same time. (Figure 8)
4. Smile upward, squeeze and hold for count of 4.
5. Contract your neck muscles and hold for another count of 4. (Figure 9)
6. Relax.
7. Repeat this exercise 8 times.

Do's and Don'ts:

DO the **Smile-up** to contract and relax the many muscles, to develop the tone and lift the tissue.

DO make this exercise a regular daily routine before breakfast and before bedtime or more often.

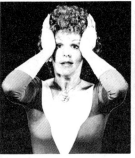
(Figure 7)

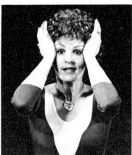
(Figure 8)

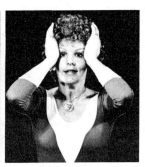
(Figure 9)

Three other poses which greatly improve the circulation and the muscle tone in the face are listed with the Day on which they are described:

Plough (Day 2, page 20)
Spread Leg Stretch Standing (Day 12, page 113)
Shoulderstand (Day 2, page 19)

13

POSE OF A CHILD

Meditation is not easily defined. It is a collective term for any number of techniques — all of them working toward the one goal of self-realization. When one Yogi was asked: "But what *do* you practise, if it is not Transcendental Meditation?" — he answered, "*Super* - Transcendental Meditation." Whatever its approach, or its name, meditation follows three distinct steps: concentration (of which a cousin is visualization), contemplation and finally, meditation. Each one of these stages needs to be fully practised before you are able to proceed or even to understand the next. No pianist has ever performed on stage without practising every one of these steps. Indeed, he is meditating whenever he practises the piano. Success comes through concentration in all fields. It is the stepping stone to infinite possibilities. Schiller said, "Genius is concentration." The reverse could be also true, because concentration is SINGLE-POINTED. A genius is rarely universal — his talent exceeds that of others in only one direction. Meditation, however, is all-enveloping.

In these fourteen days, we will approach the practice of meditation in modest little steps, up through its beginning stages. I can remember when the word 'MEDITATING' filled me with a vague fear of the unknown, the mystical. There is nothing mystical about meditation. Let us start on concentration by first becoming *aware*.

Curling Leaf   (See Figures 122, 123 — Day 14)

1. Kneel with legs together.
2. Rest your buttocks on the heels and the top of your hands on the floor, pointing back.
3. Lower your head slowly to the floor, the hands sliding gently back, palms up, to lie beside the body.
4. Rest your head on the floor on the forehead or turned to the side, and relax completely with the chest against the knees.
5. Hold for any length of time, the longer the better.

Now, let yourself go. Feel the body touching the floor, sink into it. Be completely relaxed. Be aware of your chest as it slightly moves up and down against your thighs, while you breathe regularly. Concentrate on your body rhythm through your breath. Up, down, in, out. Be aware of only your breath, follow its in-going and out-going rhythm. BE your breath! Continue as long as comfort prevails.

Day 2

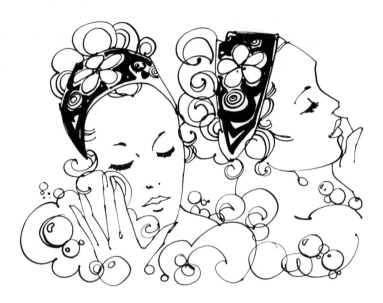

FACE — CLEANSING

What You Should Know!

— Cosmeticians vary widely in opinion on the subject of soap. Out of 12 experts, six will be for its use, six against. What everyone does agree on, however, is the *importance* of cleanliness. Since our facial muscles and skin are fed by the bloodstream — your avenues to beauty — it is of utmost importance to cleanse *inside* as well as out.
— Constipation is every person's enemy. It causes a dull, lifeless complexion, pimples, headaches, bad breath and listlessness.

What You Can Do!

1. The first step in a thorough cleansing program is to rid the facial skin and neck of the effects of pollution, greasy make-up preparations, central heating and the skin's own eliminative function.

15

2. Some experts counsel the use of an oil-based cleansing cream or cleansing milk, followed by an astringent or toning agent. Others advise following the milk with soap. Others still, advocate no cleansing lotions at all, only the soap.

3. Remember to use only very gentle upward and outward motions on the face, except for the eye area where the motion should be circular.

4. If you choose soap as your cleansing agent (as I do) opt for a clear, see-through soap gently applied with a face-cloth. Lots and lots of rinsing is a must: the famous Laszlo of New York spoke of 40 warm rinsings under running water.

5. To return the skin to its normal acid state (ph), use a few drops of apple cider vinegar in the rinse-water. My grand-mother, who, at age 79, has wonderful skin, recently told me her secret: every day she cuts up a lemon, drinks the juice and then rubs her face, hands and arms with the inside of the squeezed lemon.

6. The theory of opening and closing the pores with hot and cold water has now been largely disproved. However, steaming the face over a pot of hot water to which camomile has been added, with a towel over both head and pot, is still considered a good way to cleanse the skin through perspiration. Since this can be quite strenuous for some faces, it should be done only once a week.

7. A very effective weekly ritual is the use of a slightly abrasive cleanser which helps to clear clogged pores. Cosmetic firms give a choice of gritty creams or powders; natural meals, such as Almond Meal (see page 34 for the recipe) can be made at home.

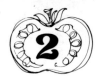

Hints to Dieter

1. Do not tell anyone, except the closest family, that you are on a diet. There is always one 'helpful' soul who says "but you don't *need* to lose weight."

2. Try to avoid dinner invitations for these two weeks.

3. Take time to make every mealtime a *visual feast;* use the best china and cutlery, napkins, candles, even flowers.

4. Knit or crochet to keep those hands busy and out of the fridge outside of meal or snack times.

5. Promise yourself the treat of a dress or a bikini for the time when you have brought your weight down. It is much cheaper in the long run than the hospital bills for illness you may incur because of overweight.

6. Go on a diet with a friend or join a diet club where the loss of face will prevent you from slipping.

7. Once you have slipped, don't consider the whole day ruined; simply eat less for the rest of that day.

8. Try not to "think food" during your diet. Do not talk about it, look at magazine pictures of it or drool over T.V. food advertisements. Tune out food, tune in culture. Read that book for which you have always meant to find time.

9. Keep a little calorie counter booklet handy to check *every* morsel you want to eat. You will be surprised at all the hidden calories.

10. When the uncontrollable appetite-urge strikes, exercise or do the Cooling Breath, to decrease your hunger pangs.

11. Use small plates and children's cutlery for your main meals.

12. Always have snackfoods (carrot sticks, cheeses, cucumbers) *ready* and prepared for quick consumption.

13. Drink a cup of bouillon half an hour before a meal to curb the appetite.

14. Chew every bit of food thoroughly, about 30 times. It not only helps your digestion and exercises the lazy facial muscles, but gives the stomach a chance to signal the brain that it is full (a process which takes about 1/2 hour).

KAREEN'S NUTRITIOUS WEIGHT LOSS DIET

MENU FOR DAY 2

Breakfast	Bowl of fresh mixed fruit: melon, berries, peaches, pineapple, grapefruit, orange, papaya or apple.
Mid-morning	250 ml. (8 oz.) vegetable juice or ½ cantaloupe.
Lunch	250 ml. (8 oz.) tomato juice 1 cup yogurt (preferably without additives and sugar, just honey)
Mid-afternoon	250 ml. (8 oz.) vegetable juice
Dinner	raw vegetable salad (as much as you like) grated carrot, beet, cabbage, green onion, chopped parsley, ½ tbsp. oil & vinegar dressing.
Before bed	1 medium apple or ½ cantaloupe

WEIGHT CONTROL

Breathing exercise for the day is the **Cooling Breath** for people suffering from a fever, wanting to quit smoking and wanting to decrease their appetite.

1. Sit comfortably in a cross-legged position, back straight.
2. Form your tongue into a trough and let it protrude slightly from the lips. Use a pencil or little finger to make your tongue round.
3. Inhale air slowly through this trough with a hissing sound.
4. Hold your breath for 1 - 5 seconds.
5. Exhale through the nostrils, pulling tummy muscles in.
6. Repeat 5 more times.

18

Do's and Don'ts:

DO this breath before you are ill, so that you know how to do it when you get a fever.

DON'T inhale too forcefully, but make it a steady, slow pull, expanding the chest and abdomen.

The Shoulderstand — presses the chin against the thyroid gland which *regulates* its function and helps to both increase and decrease weight. This pose relieves pressure on abdominal organs due to body inversion, which, in turn, regulates digestive processes, frees the body of toxins and increases the energy level.

Technique:

1. Lie on the floor, legs out-stretched, hands close by your side, palms down. Inhale.
2. Exhale, slowly lift your legs (pressing the small of the back against the floor) until they are perpendicular.
3. Press down on your hands, making them hollow or tent-like. (Figure 10)
4. Raise your buttocks and lower back and grasp yourself around the waist, with the thumbs around the front of the body. DO NOT let the elbows flare out. (Figure 11)

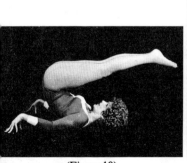 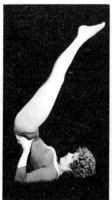 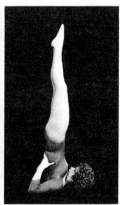

(Figure 10)   (Figure 11)   (Figure 12)

5. Straighten the legs and tuck the bottom in as much as balance permits. This is the Half Shoulderstand.

6. If you are balancing well, then grasp yourself up higher on the rib-cage and tuck your bottom in. (Figure 12)

7. Stretch your legs and point your toes. Hold the position from 10 - 60 seconds, as a beginner. Gradually work up to 3 minutes. Breathe normally throughout.

Do's and Don'ts:

DO be patient with yourself. The important thing is to be up there at all, even if it is not ramrod straight at the start.

DO NOT get alarmed if you feel slightly dizzy or heady at first. It is quite normal and can be blamed on the sudden dilation of the blood vessels.

The Plough — stimulates the thyroid gland, strengthens and firms the abdomen, as well as slimming and firming thighs and hips, and bosom; helps to decrease dowager's hump.

Technique:

1. Lie on your back on the floor, legs outstretched, arms extended by your side, palms down.

2. Exhale, slowly lift your legs by pressing the small of the back against the floor.

3. Push down on your hands, making them hollow or tent-like and raise your buttocks and lower back.(Figure 13)

4. Bring your legs over your head, attempting to touch the floor behind you with the toes, by bending at the waist. Keep your knees straight. (Figure 14)

5. Hold the position, even if your feet are nowhere near the floor, for as long as you comfortably can or up to a minute.

6. Breathe normally.

7. *Variation:* Spread your legs after you touch the floor. (Figure 15)

8. Slowly come out of the pose by bending your knees, but straighten the legs when they are perpendicular to the floor.

20

Do's and Don'ts:

DO NOT become discouraged if you can only raise your bottom a couple of inches off the floor. Simply go as far as you can, hold it there and repeat this action several times. The holding process strengthens and prepares the proper muscles for the exercise.

DO keep your knees straight throughout.

DO NOT lift your head as you lower your legs.

DO breathe normally. It will get easier with practice.

DO place your legs on a low bench behind you, if you experience a breathless sensation at first. This will pass with familiarity of the pose.

(Figure 13)

(Figure 14)

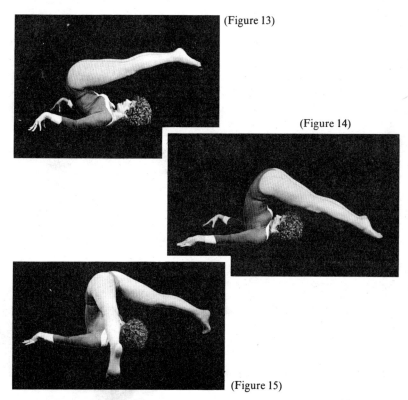

(Figure 15)

21

The Fish — stimulates the thyroid gland and strengthens the chest and bust. It is a great de-tensionizer as well as straightening the windpipe and expanding the chest for people with respiratory problems.

Technique:

1. Lie on your back, legs outstretched, arms by your side, palms down. (Figure 16). Exhale.
2. Pushing down on the elbows, raise your chest off the floor, really arching the back.
3. At the same time pull your head under until you are resting on the very top of it or as close as you can get to the crown. (Figure 17)
4. Shift your weight so that the brunt of it is being borne by the buttocks.
5. Hold the position for 5 - 60 seconds or until you start to be uncomfortable. Breathe normally.
6. Slowly come out of the asana and repeat twice more.

Do's and Don'ts:

DO put most of your body weight onto the buttocks and elbows.
DO NOT bend your legs.

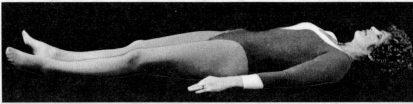

(Figure 16)

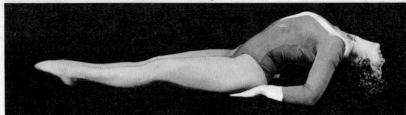

(Figure 17)

Three other poses highly recommended for Weight Control are:

Hip Bend (Day 10, page 95)
Half Locust (Day 9, page 85)
Spread Leg Stretch Standing (Day 12, page 113)

CONCENTRATION ON A TASK

The word Yoga means yoke or union. Yoga seeks to unite into one strong unit the body, soul and mind. In the untrained man these three are like oxen all trying to pull the plough in different directions. To train all three aspects of the body, yoga gives you a choice, according to temperament, of six main forms. Only half of the sixth form, Raja Yoga, is meditative. Its other half, the Hatha Yoga we practise in this book is physical. Hatha Yoga was first designed to control the body, the better to control the mind. This is done by first bringing the body to optimum organic health, and then controlling its restlessness, its bodily desires and its functions.

The purpose of meditation is to unite the concrete with the abstract, the matter with the mind, the self with the universe. Meditation has no religion. It is a turning inward of one's attentions. Try to see how your mind works. Whenever you do anything, direct all your energy into it. Meditation needs a lot of practice, but contrary to most things in life, its very practice brings its own rewards.

Start a most satisfying beginner's technique today: concentrating on a task. Let's start with dishwashing. Be totally positive in your approach to it, even if you usually dislike it. Wash the dishes with all your being! With love! Appreciate the modern facilities you have: running, hot water, soapy suds, helpful gadgets. Admire the perfection, the smoothness of each dish. Concentrate on getting everything sparkling clean. Take satisfaction in rinsing thoroughly. Work fast, yet well. Enjoy the feeling of the drying cloth against the pottery. CONCENTRATE on just washing the dishes, let no other thoughts intrude. Concentration is the first step to meditation and the first rung on the ladder of success in anything you hope to achieve.

Day 3

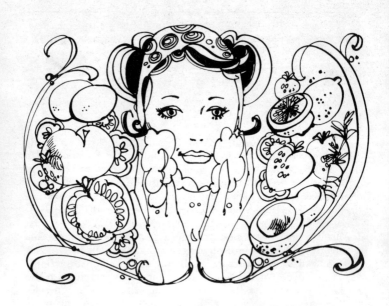

FACE — MOISTURIZING AND MASKS

What You Should Know!

— The beauty of your skin is in direct proportion to its moisture content. Skin dryness may be caused not only by the loss of the oily sebum (oily lubricant brought to the surface through tiny ducts) but also by the lack of moisture in the air.
— Moisture plumps out wrinkles.
— Good moisturizers are water, thin lotions or heavier nourishing creams.
— Showers are very useful for both face and body because they stimulate the circulation.
— An excellent beautifier is said to be a facecloth soaked in soft rain water. Cover the face with it for at least 10 minutes.

— Natural cosmetics products — good enough to eat — are enjoying a well-deserved recognition, particularly in Europe. Eggs, honey, oatmeal, cucumber, strawberries, apricots, carrots, turnips, avocados, tomatoes, lemons, milk and olive oil are all being used again as they were by the ancient Egyptians, the ladies of the French court and our own grandmothers.

What You Can Do!

1. Facial masks are the oldest form of beauty treatment known to man. They have the multiple purpose of bringing impurities to the surface and of feeding the skin.

2. **Kareen's mask:** After cleansing the skin thoroughly, apply a mask of beaten egg yolk combined with olive oil, leave on for 10 minutes, wash off gently with washcloth. This is excellent for plumping out the skin when it looks tired and drawn.

3. For a more thorough treatment before an evening out, follow step 2 with an application of cotton pads dipped in egg white — an excellent tightening mask. It can also be used most effectively by itself.

4. You can make yet another super mask by beating the egg white until stiff, then adding a teaspoon of nourishing honey.

5. A relatively new beauty treatment recommended by the heart specialist, Dr. W. Shute, whose wife and daughter have used it with great success, is the application of Vitamin E oil (start with a 100 I.U. capsule broken open) to the crows' feet around the eyes. It is also used for kitchen burns, sunburns and on scars with excellent results.

6. Consider the use of a vapourizer in your bedroom through the winter months.

7. Soap should never be left on the face longer than 20 seconds.

More Hints to Dieter

1. Never eat while standing up.

2. Never eat while watching T.V. or while at the movies.

3. Get into the habit of weighing all your food. A little kitchen scale is an excellent investment for a lifetime of weight control.

4. Try to keep your mind off food by helping other people in trouble. Even the serving of food to others, perhaps in hospitals, is personally rewarding and seems to lessen *your* need to eat.

5. The next time you feel unreasonably hungry, remind yourself that an overweight person cannot possibly be truly hungry. He merely has an appetite — in his head.

6. To lose one pound, you must have a "bank" deficit of 3500 calories. The more you weigh, the more calories you use up when you exercise and exercise has been proven to *decrease* appetite.

7. Low-calorie vegetables for in-between snacks are: celery, carrots, cucumbers, mushrooms, cauliflower, parsley, kohl-rabi, radishes, asparagus, green beans, zucchini, sauerkraut, dill pickles, spinach, red and green peppers, cabbage, green onions, lettuce. They are excellent raw in salads.

8. Keep up your diet notebook every day and record each extra peanut, lettuce leaf or "taste" while cooking.

9. Hang a picture of yourself when you were slim or a magazine picture of someone you would love to look like, on the outside of the cookie cupboard.

10. Hang the picture of a fat woman inside the refrigerator for that extra reminder *after* you have opened the door.

KAREEN'S NUTRITIOUS WEIGHT LOSS DIET

MENU FOR DAY 3

Breakfast	1 tsp. flaked yeast mixed with 1 cup orange juice 1 poached or soft-boiled egg 8 oz. (1 cup) partially skimmed milk
Mid-morning	1 tbsp. honey or ½ banana with 1 tbsp. coconut

Lunch	1 cup beet borscht*
	    or 1 cup consomme
	3 oz. (¾ cup) tuna with lemon juice
	    add: watercress or alfalfa sprouts
	        or lettuce
	6 chilled asparagus spears
	2 wheat thin crackers or rye crisps.

Mid-afternoon	1 medium apple or ½ cantaloupe
Dinner	½ cup plain yogurt* mixed with 1 tsp. honey, dredged over Fruit cup consisting of 1 orange, ½ grapefruit, and ½ banana
Bedtime snack	1 chicken breast or 1 thin slice roast beef

* See recipe section

Note:
Diet may be repeated providing the complete daily program is not altered.

NECK AND CHIN

Breathing exercise for today is the **Complete Breath**.

1. Sit in a comfortable cross-legged position or in a chair.
2. Straighten your back, which will straighten your thorax for easier breathing.
3. Inhale *slowly* through the nose, into the back of the throat, breathing deeply, consciously.
4. Take five seconds to fill the lower part of the lungs, by expanding the ribs and pushing the abdomen out.
5. Concentrate on filling the top of the lungs for the next five seconds. This will expand the chest and tighten the abdomen slightly.
6. Hold the breath for 1 - 5 seconds.
7. Exhale slowly, pulling the abdomen in until you have emptied the lungs.
8. Repeat 4 - 5 times more.

Do's and Don'ts:

DO establish a rhythmic rise and fall of your abdomen - rib cage, to promote regular breathing.

DO attempt to breathe inaudibly after you have got the knack of deep breathing.

DO NOT slump. For maximum efficiency the thorax must be straight.

DO concentrate on your breathing alone, with your eyes closed, if you wish. It serves to do the technique better but it is also a preparation for meditation.

DO push your abdomen out as you breathe in and pull the abdomen in as you breathe out.

DO give an extra snort as you exhale to rid yourself of stale waste-matter in the bottom of the lungs.

The Cat Stretch — is an excellent warm-up for any Yoga work-out; it tightens the neck and chin area, and strengthens and firms the arms.

Technique:

1. Kneel on all fours.
2. Rocking slightly back first, inhale and lower your chest in a

28

sweeping motion, trying to rest the Adam's apple on the floor. (Figure 18)

3. Hold the position for 5 seconds, with most of the weight on the arms.
4. Exhale. Return to the first position and arch the back in an upward motion rather like an angry, spitting cat. (Figure 19)
5. Hold for 5 seconds, relax.
6. Reverse the arch by pushing abdomen towards the floor and bring the head up. (Figure 20) Repeat steps 4, 5 & 6 several times.
7. Repeat steps 1, 2, 3 & 4. Now bring your right knee towards the head, and touch it if you can. Hold 5 seconds.
8. Stretch the leg out and up in back, keeping it straight. Hold. Keep the head up and arms straight. (Figure 21)
9. Return the leg slowly to the head. Hold.
10. Relax. Repeat on the other side.
11. Repeat the whole series once more.

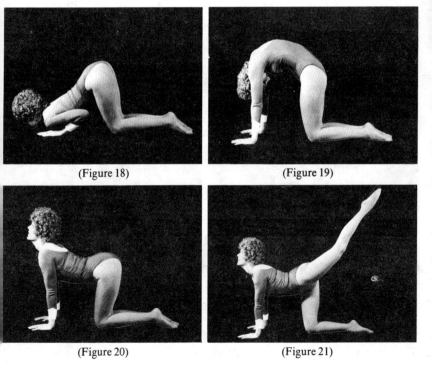

(Figure 18)   (Figure 19)

(Figure 20)   (Figure 21)

Do's and Don'ts:

DO enjoy the stretching movement of your body. Move slowly and
    with grace.

DO NOT be discouraged if you cannot get your knees to your head
    for a while. It will come.

Neck Rolls — reduce deep seated tension in the neck area, relieve
    stiff neck and often headaches. They help to get rid of double
    chin and necklines with enough repetitions.

Technique:

1. Sit at a table, back straight.
2. Place your elbows directly in front of you on the table. All of
   the lower arms should be touching each other, from elbow to
   inner wrists. (Figure 22)
3. Form a cup of the hands and place the head in the middle of
   the cup.
4. Leaving the wrists together, slowly turn the head to the
   RIGHT until the LEFT side of the chin is lying in the RIGHT
   palm. The LEFT palm will be supporting the head over the
   LEFT ear. (Figure 23)
5. Slowly start to push the chin to the RIGHT with the RIGHT
   hand, as though you wanted to hoist the head off. Hold the
   pressure for a few seconds. Release. Repeat on other side.

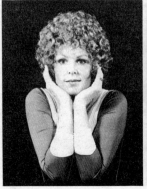
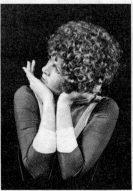
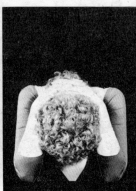

(Figure 22)   (Figure 23)   (Figure 24)

6.   Place both hands with fingers interlaced on back of the head. Push down. Hold the pressure as you push back with your head. (Figure 24)
7.   Release after a few seconds and repeat 2 more times.

___

Apple-Biting — is an excellent way to tighten the neck and chin areas and to "lubricate" the jaw joints.

Technique:

1.   Start by imagining a red, juicy apple hanging just above your head.
2.   Slowly raise your head, keeping your mouth closed until you are looking up at the ceiling. (Figure 25)
3.   Open your mouth as wide as you can and reach for the apple, keeping the arms and shoulders down. (Figure 26)
4.   Pull on the muscles of the throat and neck, then relax, bending head forward. (Figure 27)
5.   Repeat the whole exercise at least 8 times every night.

Do's and Don'ts:

DO stretch the bottom jaw as far as possible for maximum benefits to the neck.
DO pull, pull, pull towards that apple to tone the chin.

Other poses which work on the neck/chin are:
Cobra (Day 6, page 59)
Fish (Day 2, page 22)
Crow (Day 6, page 58)

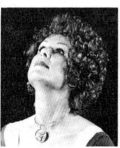
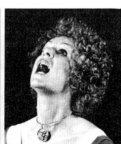
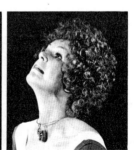

(Figure 25)   (Figure 26)   (Figure 27)

31

THE SENSE SEALER

Most of us are tyrannized by our senses. We are slaves to our thoughts, our fears and our desires. What a blessed relief it would be sometimes, to become senseless, thoughtless. Meditation aims toward this. Swami Shyam Acharya calls it "creating a situation of stillness". He goes on: "Meditation concerns those who are desirous of improving their physical environments, their family matters and the affairs vitally concerned with the welfare of mankind. To them I say that they should shift their attention from the outer aspect of life towards the inner man who wants to grow and fulfill himself at any cost, under any circumstances... there must be no wastage of energy by way of scattered thoughts." The **Sense Sealer** helps you to gather yourself inward by manually shutting the senses for you. Thus a beginner does not have to dissipate energy in doing so by strength of will. In this breathing pose, concentrate again on the in and out flow of your breath. Do not let yourself get annoyed if other thoughts intrude, simply shift the attention back to the breath. Continue as long as comfort permits.

Sense Sealer

1. Sit in a comfortable cross-legged position, spine straight.
2. Raise your arms so that the elbows are at shoulder height and place the hands on either side of the nose.
3. Now close the eyes, look upwards and place the index and middle fingers on the eyelids.
4. The ring fingers now gently push against the nostrils, the opening an oval rather than a round shape. The little fingers rest somewhere below the nostrils.
5. Now place the thumbs against the earholes and apply gentle pressure on ears and eyes.
6. Breathe normally and concentrate on the ebb and flow of your breath. Think of nothing else.
7. Perform only 3 - 4 breaths at first, increasing this by one breath a week until you are doing it for 5 - 10 minutes.

The **Sense Sealer** can be considered one of the bridges between Hatha Yoga and Meditation. It is designed to still the mind, to turn the gaze inward — for peace is to be found nowhere else. Normally, our senses keep us chained to darkness as each one tempts us to follow its desires. Spiritual enlightenment can only come when we are desireless.

Day 4

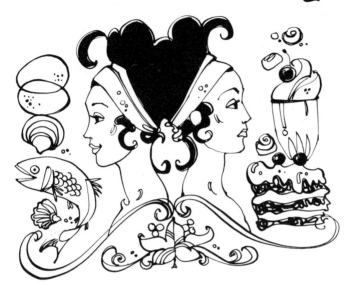

FACE – PROBLEMS

What You Should Know!

— The most common skin problems are pimples, blackheads and red blotches.
— Acne in the teenager is caused by the combined stresses of rapid growth, inadequate diet, social pressures and emotional problems.
— In adults, poor diet and emotional stress are the villains.
— Skin problems should always be taken to a doctor or dermatologist first, but nutritional information should be considered also.

What You Can Do!

1. Be scrupulously clean. Pores become plugged by surface dirt or by sebum, which hardens and turns black when it reaches the air. When it then becomes infected, a pimple results. Oily skin can benefit from a cool fennel tea solution.
2. Sharply lower your carbohydrate intake, particularly of sugar products, soft drinks, and spicy, greasy foods.

33

3. Add Vitamin A (25,000 I.U.) and E (which protects the A) to your diet. When an A deficiency exists, cells below the skin die and slough off, plugging the oil-sacs, making the skin so dry that it itches.
4. Increase your intake of zinc, found in egg yolks, meat and seafoods.
5. Some doctors advise applying iodine to an erupting pimple.
6. Use a heated honey mask to draw out impurities.
7. Use a gritty cleanser, such as the almond cleanser, to get skin thoroughly clean.
8. For blotchy skin, the apple cider vinegar rinse (1 part vinegar to 8 parts water) works wonders.
9. Try to calm down the nerves with extra calcium and pantothenic acid (a B-vitamin) in your diet.
10. Don't punish your skin for the anger you feel against the pimples, by squeezing them too hard.

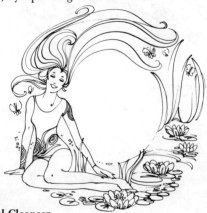

Almond Meal Cleanser
(Excellent for teenagers and people with oily skin)

— Use almonds without skins.
   (To remove skins, drop into boiling water; cool, remove skin and leave to dry overnight.)
— Grind almonds to a fine meal in blender or coffee grinder.
— Moisten face and rub small quantity all over the face; work into problem areas around the nose and other folds.
— Rinse off with lukewarm water.
— Blot dry.

Sprouting for Good Health

If you were given the choice of only one food to eat for the rest of your life, you would be well advised to choose sprouts. They come from the "seeds of life" and have all the potential energy and food stored for the growing plant. Use sprouts in salads (potato, spinach), on their own with dressing, in soups and casseroles. You can sprout alfalfa seeds, mung beans, mustard seed, lentils, wheat, fenugreek and sunflowers. Sprouts contain large amounts of Vitamins B, C and E. When seeds sprout, their vitamin content increases greatly to give us a most inexpensive source of natural vitamins. (Sunflower seeds and pumpkin seeds are delicious when sprouted for only one day and served in salad).

How to Sprout your own:

1. Let the seeds stand in water for one day. Drain.
2. Rinse in lukewarm water once or twice a day, drain immediately afterwards.
3. Keep in a dark cupboard or corner.
4. Glass jars with cheese cloth or fine screen across the opening are easy to use, care for, drain and clean.

Rules for good Sprouting:

1. Always keep the sprouts moist, never dry, never too wet. Handle them carefully — remember they are little plants and are *alive.*
2. Keep them warm. This makes them grow faster. (The warmer they are kept the more often they must be rinsed to prevent them from getting dry).
3. Alternate: Use a colander lined with paper towelling and cover the seeds with another wet sheet. Keep these moist with a daily drenching. The colander will take care of the draining.

KAREEN'S NUTRITIOUS WEIGHT LOSS DIET

MENU FOR DAY 4.

Breakfast	½ grapefruit
	¼ cup crunchy granola* type cereal with 2% milk (4 oz.)
	or Pineapple Blender Drink:
	1 cup pineapple juice
	1 tbsp. non-instant skim milk powder
	1 tsp. yeast powder
	1 tsp. raw wheat germ
	1 egg
Mid-morning	1 tbsp. peanut butter or ½ cup peanuts.
Lunch	Fruit salad with cottage cheese:
	½ banana, ½ apple, ½ orange, pineapple cubes, 2 tbsp. cottage cheese
	1 cup 2% milk
Mid-afternoon	10 almonds
Dinner	Alfalfa sprouts,
	or lettuce
	or 1 cup water cress
	with 1 medium tomato sliced
	½ tbsp. oil & vinegar dressing
	4 oz. beef liver, broiled.
Bedtime snack	1 banana
	or ½ cantaloupe

* See recipe section

POSTURE

Breathing exercise for the day is called **Mountain**.

1. Sit in a comfortable cross-legged position, the back straight.
2. Bring the palms of both hands together in front of your chest, as if praying.
3. Pressing the palms firmly together, inhale, expanding the rib cage, and slowly stretch the arms above the head. Stretch the finger-tips toward the ceiling in a tremendous stretch. Hold for 5 seconds.
4. Slowly bring the hands down, exhaling.
5. Relax.

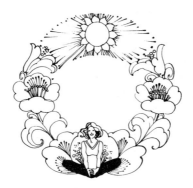

The Arm and Leg Stretch — promotes good balance and firms and stretches the front of the body.

Technique:

1. Stand straight, heels together, toes slightly pointed outward.
2. Raise your right arm slowly so that it stands out at an angle but the hand is above the head. The elbows are straight.
3. Bend your left leg at the knee, bringing it close to the buttocks, and shift your body weight onto the right foot.
4. Grasp your left foot with your left hand. (Figure 28)
5. Bend backward from the waist, at the same time pulling on the foot and moving the right arm as far back as balancing permits. Let the head drop back. (Figure 29)
6. Hold this position 5 seconds at the start, increasing the time at 5 seconds a week.

37

7. If you have no trouble with balance, try to tilt your body forward while you hold the position described. (Figure 30)

8. Repeat on the other side and perform the asana three times on each side.

Do's and Don'ts:

DO simple balancing exercises such as the **Tree** first, if you have difficulty keeping your balance.

DO concentrate fiercely, it will help you to keep your balance better.

DO move slowly when going into and coming out of the **Arm and Leg Stretch,** as in all Yoga exercises.

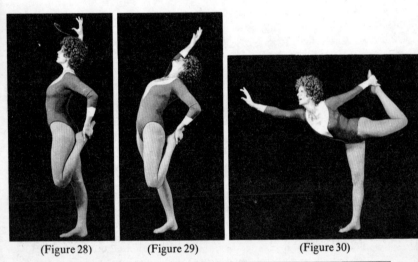

(Figure 28)   (Figure 29)   (Figure 30)

The Dog Stretch — acts as an energizer, makes legs and ankles shapely, relieves stiffness and tension in the neck and shoulders and firms the bust.

Technique:

1. Lie on your stomach, hands beside the shoulders, fingers pointing forward. (Figure 31)

2. Tuck the toes under, EXHALE and push down on your hands lifting the body in a straight line as in an Army push-up.

38

3. When the arms are straight, bend the body at the waist and push the bottom up, shifting the weight onto the feet. (Figure 32)
4. Move the head toward the feet and place the very top of the head on the floor. (Figure 33)
5. Keep the knees straight and push the heels toward the floor.
6. Stretch the back and keep the elbows straight, sliding the hands forward, if necessary.
7. Hold the pose, breathing normally 15 - 60 seconds.
8. EXHALE, lower the body to the floor, and relax.
9. Repeat twice more, if you did not hold the pose for very long.

Do's and Don'ts:

DO bend the elbows somewhat, if it is necessary in order to bring the head to the floor.

DO try to do this pose in your bare feet, so that you won't slide.

DO attempt this pose from an all-fours position at first, if your arms are too weak for the push-up motion.

DO push your heels towards the floor.

DO NOT bend the knees.

DO remember that the **Dog Stretch** is a very advanced pose and as such will take some time to master.

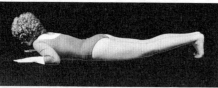

(Figure 31)

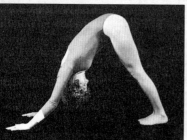

(Figure 32)

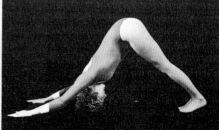

(Figure 33)

The Posture Clasp—is excellent for improving posture and rounded shoulders. It eases tension in the shoulders as it oils the joints and exercises the muscles in the upper back.

Technique:

1. Kneel resting on the heels, legs together, back straight.
2. Bring your left hand behind your back, palm facing out and try to wriggle it up your back as far as it will go. (Figure 34)
3. Lift your right hand straight up and bend it at the elbow, bringing the hand to the centre of the back. This pose is also called the **Cow Head** pose because of the elbow sticking up to look like a horn.

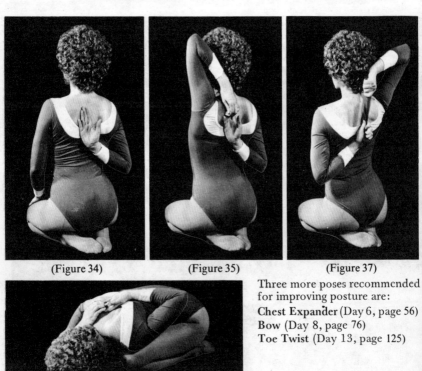

(Figure 34)   (Figure 35)   (Figure 37)

(Figure 36)

Three more poses recommended for improving posture are:
Chest Expander (Day 6, page 56)
Bow (Day 8, page 76)
Toe Twist (Day 13, page 125)

40

4. Try to get the two hands close enough together to interlock the fingers, by gently inching them together.
5. Hold the position for 10 - 30 seconds and try a gentle upward pull with the right hand, then a downward pull with the left. (Figure 35)
6. Repeat on the other side and twice more on both sides.
7. You will find that one side is much more flexible than the other. Concentrate on the stiffer one.
8. Variation: After you have mastered the Posture Clasp, try bending forward to touch your forehead to the floor. (Figure 36)

Do's and Don'ts:

DO keep your back straight and you will have better success.
DO NOT strain beyond a point of comfort
DO use a kerchief if your fingers are too far apart. (Figure 37)

LEARNING TO CONTROL THE THOUGHTS

How often do we lie in bed, unable to sleep because one worrisome thought chases the next like restless bats in a belfry? We'd give anything to be able to interrupt this flow of thought, to drop off abruptly into sleep. However, often even this sleep is restless as we twitch and turn under the influence of our nervous system. "Super Silence" is not possible, even at night, without practice. One must learn through meditation, not to still all thought — an utter impossibility for the untrained Western mind — but to cut down on the volume of it. How, where and when does one practise meditation? There is no mystery about this — simply be comfortable, watch the thoughts and BE. Assume a basic meditation pose, where all the senses are occupied or excluded so that they will not distract us. Sit in a quiet, peaceful, well-aired part of the house. It should have good seating, where the back is reasonably straight, the feet are up and the head can be supported. Try to choose a quiet time, but accept the fact that this is a noisy world and don't let yourself be irritated by the odd noise. Burn some incense or wear a perfume to have the sense of smell satisfied. Close your eyes. Hold a flower between your folded hands so that they will not restlessly search for occupation. Set a clock to go off in 5, 10, 15 or 30 minutes — as long as you feel you can sit still — so that you do not have to think about time.

Now let's sit back and be witnesses to ourselves. Let the thoughts stream by. Watch, be aware, but DO NOT BECOME INVOLVED! Above all, do not wrangle with negative thoughts, with worries. So often people are very careful about the company they keep — undesirable characters are kept out of the house. But they show no discrimination in what bad company they let inside their mind: negative, useless, foolish, and perhaps even malicious thoughts. Let's try to weed them out, now. Observe the never-ending flow of thought, connected by association, but ease out the bad ones. This will cut down on their number considerably, and that is the beginning of restful meditation.

Day 5

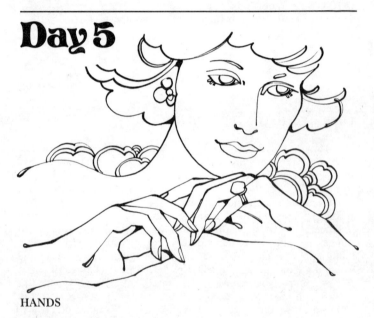

HANDS

What You Should Know!

— Your hands have the same personality traits as the skin on your face.
— All rules concerning it, particularly nutritional ones, also apply to your hands.
— The hands are also the only truly unprotected, indisguisable part of your body. They give your age away.

— From prose and poetry we know that people notice our hands more than we would suspect, judging a woman's beauty by her overall appearance, not just her face.

— Bulging veins can be made to disappear by making a habit of holding the hands up; liver spots can be made to fade with natural bleaching agents or by taking extra Vitamin B-2; rough and large-pored skin can be repaired with nourishing creams and lotions.

What You Can Do!

1. Natural bleaching agents for liver spots are buttermilk left on to dry, or wheat germ oil gently rubbed in for 3 - 4 minutes.
2. To take stains, such as nicotine, off fingers or nails, rub them with a raw potato or a slice of lemon.
3. One of the most beautifying agents for both hands and face is a mixture of glycerine and rosewater in equal parts. Apply this before bedtime and then wear a pair of slightly large white cotton gloves all night. Mayonnaise is also effective, especially for gardeners' hands.
4. Make a habit of keeping a lanolin-based hand lotion near both the kitchen and the bathroom sink and use it after every washing; don't neglect the arm and elbow.
5. One of the most terrible drying agents on hands is water. Never let the water on either your face or your hands dry by itself.
6. Try to get used to rubber gloves in the kitchen — after all, surgeons do the most delicate operations with them.
7. Put your elbows in two squeezed grapefruit or lemon halves and lean on them for 15 minutes, perhaps while reading a book. Then apply a cream. Scrub both elbows and knees with a nailbrush or a pumice-stone in the shower, often.
8. Do you have cold hands? Poor circulation can be improved with 400 - 800 international units of vitamin E. (Step up the dosage slowly — it's said to be excellent for your heart). Massage hands from the fingertips to the wrists with a deep, one-way stroke.
9. A woman is immediately more beautiful if she moves gracefully, even with her hands.

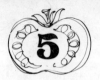

YOGA NUTRITION

The simplest definition of YOGA NUTRITION is 'food unchanged from the natural form.' The farther away we get from the natural state of food, the more knowledgeable we must be about what foods we should eat. Too many foods are over-refined, sometimes to preserve them for longer shelf-life and sometimes for 'better' taste, but in the process we are deprived of many useful nutrients. If food is refined (as are white flour, white sugar, white rice and noodles) it becomes automatically fattening because the body cannot derive nutrients from it and therefore stores it as fat. Our digestive system was designed to prepare for periods of hunger. With modern food storage, however, it is no longer necessary to put on fat, like a bear, for long winter months. Instead, means of preserving have been devised. Some of these are less damaging than others: drying fruit and vegetables delays any decomposition which may take place; grains and seeds are always dehydrated for storage; freezing is an excellent method of storage so long as it is done only once. However, by putting additives and preservatives into food in order to keep it for the future, we are not only changing the chemical structure of the original food, we are also introducing unnecessary elements into our diet. The most glaring examples are the use of sugar in preserving fruit and vegetables and the excessive quantities of salt in preserving meat as sausages. Sodium is necessary, especially during hot weather, but it must always be in balance with potassium. This mineral helps to release water from the body by releasing sodium from the cells. However, too much of it can also cause a sodium deficiency.

It quickly becomes evident that, in the body, everything is in balance and interdependent. Let me give you some interesting examples: The healing qualities of Vitamin A are doubled if Vitamin E is also taken; Lecithin helps Vitamins A, D, E, K, and fat to be carried and absorbed in the body; Vitamin D is the catalyst of the whole calcium family; PABA (a B-Vitamin) is destroyed by sulfa drugs; magnesium should be taken in conjunction with calcium, and potassium; iron destroys Vitamin E and the two should be taken 12 hours apart. The need for the B-vitamins increases in proportion to the amount of alcohol and coffee being drunk. On very hot days, when B-vitamins are lost through perspiration, and when you drink large amounts of liquids, the need for these vitamins is tremendously increased.

Do's and Don'ts:

DO make sure that your body is straight from the shoulders down, by placing yourself an arm's length from the wall.

DO push hard, in resistance to the movement, so that the sinews in the arms and fingers stand out.

Rest and breathe normally between each exercise if you wish. Keep in mind that if you have recently lost weight or if you intend to lose it, the baggy look is especially obvious on the upper arms.

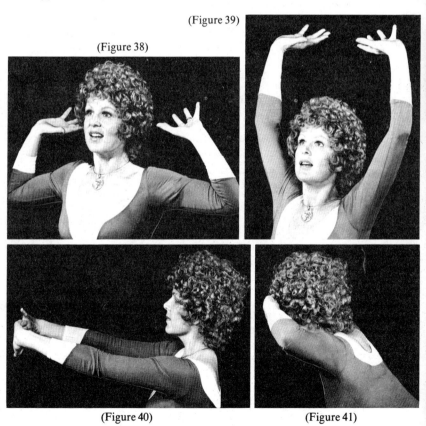

(Figure 39)

(Figure 38)

(Figure 40)

(Figure 41)

The Flower — eases the pain of arthritis and loosens stiff fingers and keeps hands looking younger and the fingers very flexible.

Technique:

1. Sit in a comfortable cross-legged position.
2. Make your hands into tight fists, squeezing hard. (Figure 42)
3. Now visualize that your hand is a flower early in the morning and ever so gently and slowly start to open the hands, resisting all the while. (Figure 43)
4. Bend the fingers all the way back. (Figure 44)
5. Reverse the motion and close the hands slowly. The movement must be resisted so that the sinews in the back of the hand stand out.
6. Relax the fingers by moving or shaking them rapidly.
7. Next, with fingers spread apart, press each finger, separately, hard against the palm, holding for 2 seconds each.
8. Repeat the whole series of exercises twice more.

Do's and Don'ts:

DO the exercises in warm water or oil and you will find a painful effort made much easier with the same benefits.

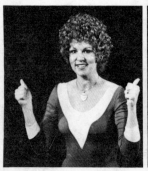

(Figure 42)   (Figure 43)   (Figure 44)

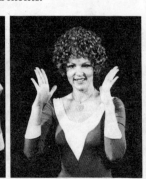

Three other poses recommended for strengthening arms and wrists are:

Crow (Day 6, page 58)
Cobra (Day 6, page 59)
Dog Stretch (Day 4, page 38)

The Finger Drill — massages the joints and keeps them flexible.

Technique:

1. With the right hand, take firm hold of your index finger of your relaxed left hand. (Figure 45)
2. Shake, pinch, and roll between your fingers, the first knuckle.
3. Move to the middle joint and repeat the massage and move the finger in circle in a clockwise manner and the reverse. (Figure 46)
4. Manipulate the last knuckle and tip of the finger in the same way.
5. Move to the middle finger and repeat steps 2, 3, & 4.
6. Repeat with ring finger, baby finger and thumb before moving to the left hand.

Do's and Don'ts:

DO enjoy the more supple joints and surprise of more pliable hands.

DO repeat this exercise on a regular daily basis to maintain healthy hands.

DO NOT worry about "cracking your fingers" — you cannot do any harm.

(Figure 45)   (Figure 46)

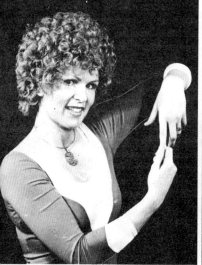
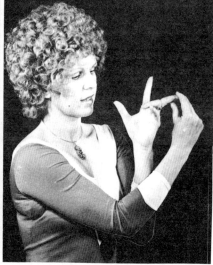

The Inclined Plane — strengthens the arms and wrists by carrying the weight of the body. Firms bosom, hips & buttocks.

Technique:

1. Sit, legs together and outstretched.
2. Lean back slightly and place the hands straight down from the shoulders, fingers pointing forward on the floor. (Figure 47) EXHALE, push down on the hands and lift the buttocks off the floor.
3. Dig the heels in and push the hips up as much as possible, arching the back. Let the head fall back. (Figure 48)
4. Hold for 10 - 60 seconds breathing normally, letting the hands and feet carry the weight.
5. EXHALE, lower the hips to the floor and relax.

(Figure 47)

Variation:

1. Repeat steps 1 - 3 above.
4. Slowly raise the right leg as high as it will go. (Figure 49)
5. Hold for 10 - 30 seconds.
6. Repeat on the other side.

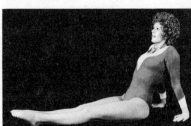

(Figure 48)

Do's and Don'ts:

DO make sure that the whole sole of the foot is resting on the floor, once the pose is achieved.

DO concentrate on the benefits, not the difficulties of the pose, while holding it.

DO distribute the body weight evenly between the hands and feet.

DO stretch the neck backward as much as possible, letting the head hang.

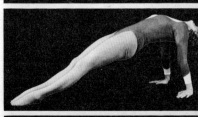

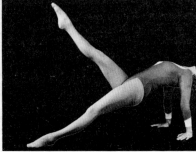

(Figure 49)

CANDLE GAZING

Meditation is a thinking process — the continuous flow of thought on one subject. Meditation is a state of mind. It can be either conscious or unconscious. We all have felt a momentary feeling of bliss, of searing beauty, of supreme desirelessness, a shiver down the spine, sudden tears in the eyes; we may have been terribly moved by a picture, a poem, a piece of music, sexual love. But this feeling always lasted only a moment, it was unconscious. The Yogi works towards a *continual* state of such bliss. This is conscious meditation.

Concentration, on the other hand, is a holding still of the mind's attention on one object. Up to now, we have practised at the kindergarten level of meditation. We have prepared for concentration by becoming aware, by watching, by being. Now is the time to start the first level of concentration. The Yogi tries to stop the restless workings of the mind, to train it to become steady (one-pointed), by consciously turning his attention onto one object. Lighting a candle is an excellent way of achieving this. Sit in a basic meditation posture, comfortable, with a straight spine. Light a candle on a low table in front of you and fix your gaze on the flame only. Look steadily at it without letting your gaze wander, but do not stare. Breathe regularly, looking at the flame for about a minute. Now close your eyes and try to visualize the light in the darkness. It should be just as clear with the eyes closed as when they are open. If you cannot see the impression of the flame clearly or if it fades quickly, open the eyes again for another long look. Repeat this exercise until you can hold the vision of the light for long periods. This might take several days, but do not be impatient with yourself or force the issue. It will come in your own good time.

Day 6

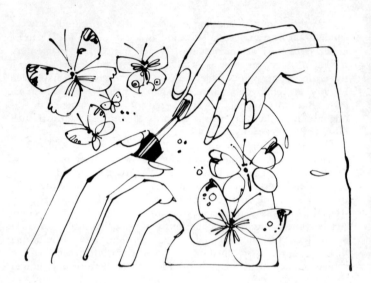

NAILS – PROBLEMS, SUPPLEMENTS

What You Should Know!

- Your nails are a dead, horny substance, largely made up of protein, which was alive while inside the finger.
- It consists of three separate layers which are glued together by an oily liquid. When this dries out, we get splitting, peeling nails.
- We know now that poor nails are due to a combination of cold weather, poor nutrition and lack of exercise (the nails seem to deteriorate and form more slowly in the winter months).
- Maintaining good nails requires knowledgeable care from the inside and the outside, but rebuilding nails is a slow process. Even when the diet is radically changed and supplemented, it takes at least six months to see any results.
- With the nails, the inner care is considerably more important than the outer care.

What You Can Do!

1. An old, though incomplete, remedy has always been the taking of flavourless gelatin. Gelatin is not a complete protein, but it becomes one when taken in milk or bouillon. An even better substitute is Japanese seaweed, called Nori, which keeps the nails from becoming brittle and is an excellent energy food with many other benefits.

2. Brittle nails which show marked longitudinal ridging tell you that you are in need of extra iron. Growing children and women need it more than men, generally speaking, and it is one of North America's greatest deficiencies; but men with a bleeding ulcer should be getting extra doses, too.

3. Vitamin A deficiency, too, shows itself by peeling and ridging.

4. A very good beauty treatment consists of heated wheat germ oil, in which the nails are soaked for 3 - 4 minutes, then massaged to encourage absorption. (Refrigerate, for re-use, as wheat germ oil quickly goes rancid).

5. The pearly nail polishes last longer but are considerably more drying than the plain ones.

6. If you have brittle nails, try the "strength through thickness" principle by careful use of nail polishes. Experiment with different brands to see which lasts longest on you; clean the nails with a non-oily polish remover just before applying the polish; let the polish dry properly (for at least 20 minutes); apply several layers, within a hairbreadth width of the cuticle; apply a quick dab of hard top coat every morning.

7. Your toe nails should never be cut in the corners, to prevent ingrowing toenail.

6

What is a Calorie?

A calorie is a unit of measurement for the amount of *heat* energy produced, when the food goes through the digestion processes. It is not a food in itself. However, the various foods yield differing amounts of heat when eaten. This explains the need for a calorie counter. Even then, the calories listed are not totally reliable. Individual powers of digestion, constipation, fatigue, stress and the vigor with which you apply yourself to any activity, all influence your personal caloric expenditure.

Normally, one should take in 2000 - 3000 calories to produce enough energy for a day's work. To gain one pound you must 'over-eat' by 3500 calories; to lose it, whether in one day or one month, you must eat 3500 calories less than your usual amount over that given period. But, a dieter should constantly remind himself that one could really speak of two types of calories: the empty, usually delicious ones and the laden with food value ones. The first are immediately stored as fat, the second are soaked up by the body as water by a sponge. The first may be a sugary lemon meringue pie (sugar is three to five times as fattening as flour products), the second could be a banana, for example. The ingredients of the pie are refined to the point of having been deprived of all nutrient value, while the banana consists of energy-giving natural fruit sugars.

It follows that the fruit cannot be fattening, since the body can immediately use its elements. Therefore, nuts are not fattening if taken as meals in themselves and not before a huge dinner; nor are oils. These last have a definite slimming value: they release water from the cells and actually help to burn off fat in the tissue.

You should also know that fatigue interferes with proper digestion. Rest, before you eat. Constipation causes the bloodstream and the liver to become polluted from gases, acids and alcohol left in the colon for long periods of time. Eat less or eat only bulk foods when you are constipated. Let the well-being of your body be your guide, not the calories. Watch and observe yourself. If you are not digesting certain raw foods well, then parboil them slightly first. Eat only what you can digest. The best diet in the world is useless if you can't digest it. And don't change your eating habits too rapidly. Our digestive juices are adapted to the foods we and our parents have eaten. The pattern can be changed, but this takes time. A fit and energetic body will

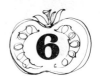

always follow good nutrition, if you help your body to use food economically, not wastefully. Then the calorie loses its importance and 'loaded' food becomes your guide.

KAREEN'S NUTRITIOUS WEIGHT LOSS DIET

MENU FOR DAY 6

Breakfast
2 tsp. flaked yeast mixed with
1 cup orange juice
2 eggs scrambled with milk and ½ pat of butter

Mid-morning
1 banana
  or ½ cantaloupe

Lunch
1 cup consomme
  or 8 oz. tomato or vegetable juice
salad of watercress, alfalfa sprouts, chopped green onions, 1 medium tomato, and 1 tbsp. hulled sunflower seeds with ½ tbsp. French dressing
  or   Orange Blender Drink:
    1 cup orange juice
    1 tsp. vanilla soy flour
    or 2 tsp. powdered yeast
    1 egg

Mid-afternoon
1 tbsp. peanut butter
  or ½ cup peanuts

Dinner
1 cup alfalfa sprouts or watercress
  or ¼ head lettuce, 1 medium tomato
seasoned with ½ tbsp. oil and vinegar dressing
½ medium baked potato
½ pat butter
3 oz. roast beef
  or 1 chicken breast

Bedtime snack
1 slice whole wheat toast spread lightly with butter and honey
  or 1 muffin (soy or wheat germ*) with ½ pat butter

* See Recipe Section

BOSOM

Today's breathing exercise is **The Alternate Nostril Breath I** to relax your body and to overcome anxiety or insomnia.

1. Sit in a comfortable cross-legged position, back straight.
2. Raise your RIGHT hand and place your RIGHT thumb, against your RIGHT nostril, closing it off.
3. Inhale deeply and slowly through the LEFT nostril to the count of four or as long as you can.
4. Exhale through the same nostril for a count of four or as long as the inhalation.
5. Concentrate on completely emptying the lungs.
6. Repeat three to four times remembering to fill the bottom, middle and top of the lungs.
7. Now change sides by closing off the LEFT nostril with your RIGHT ringfinger and follow directions 3 to 6 breathing and exhaling through the right nostril.

The Chest Expander — builds the bust for ladies and expands the chest for men. As well as acting as a quick energizer, it is an excellent way to relieve tension in the neck and shoulders.

Technique:

1. Stand straight, feet slightly apart and bring arms forward, palms together. (Figure 50)
2. Inhale, bring the arms behind the back in a wide circling motion, knifing the shoulder blades together. Clasp the hands.
3. Letting your head fall back, bend backward as far as you comfortably can, pushing the pelvis forward. Exhale.
4. Inhale, push the clasped hands up toward your head and hold this position for 5 seconds. (Figure 51)
5. Now, staying in the same position, exhale, bend slowly forward from the waist, letting the head hang down. Let your body weight pull you down, but do not jerk or bounce.
6. Hold this position for 5 - 30 seconds and keep pushing the hands up towards the head. (Figure 52) Breathe normally.
7. Inhale, straighten slowly, relax, and then repeat twice more.

Do's and Don'ts:

DO it often if you are concerned about your bustline.
DON'T close your eyes, in order to keep your balance better.

Three other poses recommended for strengthening the pectoral muscles are:

Bow (Day 8, page 76)
Inclined Plane (Day 5, page 50)
Arm Push (Day 5, page 46)

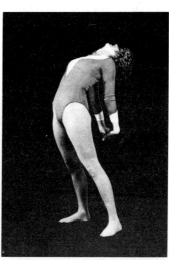

(Figure 51)

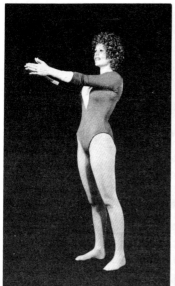

(Figure 50)

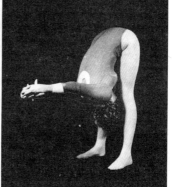

(Figure 52)

The Crow — strengthens and develops the pectoral muscles of the bustline, firms the abdomen.

Technique:

1. Squat on the heels, feet about 15 cm. (6 in.) apart (or together, for advanced students).
2. With the arms against the inside of the knees, rise onto the toes and bend slightly forward. (Figure 53)
3. Place the hands on the floor in front of you, the thumbs about 6" apart, the fingers spread and slightly pointed towards each other.
4. Now press the area of the arms just above the elbow against the side of the knee. Bring the bottom up. (Figure 54)
5. EXHALE, bend forward, bringing the face closer to the floor and gently lift the toes off, pressing the elbows against the knees. (Figure 55)
6. Try to straighten the arms as much as possible and balance on the hands breathing normally for 5 - 20 seconds.
7. EXHALE, lower the toes and relax. Repeat twice more.

Do's and Don'ts:

DO use a pillow on the floor in front of you to give you confidence.
DO keep the toes of one foot poised to help you with your balance.
DO be sure to press the area just above the elbows against the side of the knee just above the fleshy part.

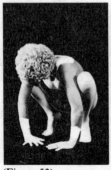 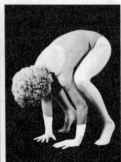 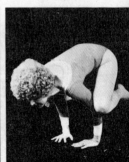

(Figure 53)   (Figure 54)   (Figure 55)

58

The Cobra — develops the pectoral muscles of the bust as it stretches and realigns the spinal column.

Technique:

1. Lie on your stomach, hands by your side, feet together.
2. Bring the hands, palms down, under the shoulders, a shoulder's width apart. (Figure 56)
3. Inhale, lift your head SLOWLY, looking up at the ceiling.
4. When the head is up as far as it will go, and only then, lift the upper shoulders and back, making the muscles of the back do most of the work, rather than the hands.
5. Continue lifting the trunk until you can go no further and still keep the pubic area on the floor. There should be a good arch in the lower spine, but the arms need not be straight. (Figure 47) Hold.

(Figure 56)

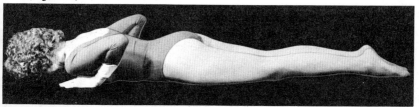

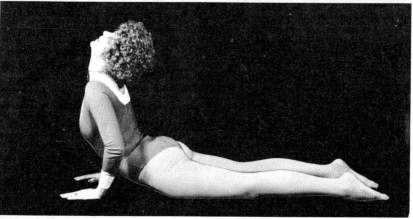

(Figure 57)

6   Exhale, slowly come out of the **Cobra** position, feeling the action of each vertebra rolling against the next, and leaving your head up to the very last.

7.   Repeat twice more, breathe normally while holding.

Do's and Don'ts:

DO make sure that your eyes look upward in their sockets throughout going into, holding and coming out of the exercise. Be aware of and enjoy the slow movement of your spine, the vertebra-by-vertebra massage.

APPLE

One of the beautiful aspects of Yoga is its flexibility. This is felt not just in its physical postures, but in the philosophical aspect as well. It is a tremendous comfort to read in the Yoga writings, that one must not force a stage of development. There is a time of ripeness, of readiness, in all things. The apple does not fall from the tree while it is still green. When it is ripe, it falls, and only then. This must be true of your approach to meditation. If you have tried concentration conscientiously and it seems impossible, simply consider it premature for you to go on to visualization or to contemplation, as yet. Persist gently in your efforts on *your* level of development. Meditation, or its steps, are a highly individual thing, concerning the individual alone. He must be on a certain level of awareness. He must not wish to master this technique for personal gain, but for his enlightenment, or he will fail. Our next step, a brother of concentration, is visualization.

Take an apple. Do with it as you did with the candle. Look at it, close your eyes, try to see it in your mind. But now, go one step further. Ponder upon the apple — its texture, its smell, its colour, its shape, its taste. Think of the many uses an apple can be put to; think of how it grew from the seed to a tree, from the tree to the fruit; the processes it went through before it reached the market. Think everything and anything about the apple, but ONLY of things connected with apples. If other thoughts persist in intruding, if association takes you off on another train of thought, gently remind yourself: the Apple.

Day 7

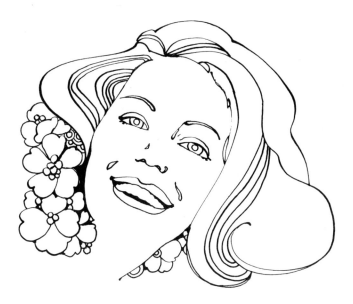

TEETH

What You Should Know!

— If you have no cavities, no removed teeth and if they are all uniform, with regular spacing, then you are a one-in-a-million person. Most of us have our fair share of fillings, dentures, crooked teeth and impacted wisdom teeth.
— Dental problems are peculiar to the "civilized" world. All the primitive societies, from the meat-eating Eskimos to the bean and corn-eating South American Indians, have excellent teeth, which deteriorate immediately when processed foods come their way.
— 99% of the body's calcium goes to the teeth and bones; 98% of North American tooth decay is caused by eating too much sugar.
— Paradoxically, the craving for sweets is caused by a nutritional deficiency in the body and can be made to disappear when the blood sugar level is kept high through foods such as protein and fats.

61

— Calcium is also an excellent nerve relaxer, so that it quietens both a menopausal mother and her growing teenager while ensuring better teeth to both of them. Remember, a dazzling smile beautifies even a plain face.

What You Can Do!

1. Exercise the teeth by eating sunflower seeds (which contain not only high quality protein but many other important nutrients) and plenty of raw salads and vegetables.

2. To keep the circulation and therefore the teeth healthy, rub the gums with your fingers.

3. Make regular visits to your dentist (modern procedure is quite painless) and ask him to instruct you in the use of dental floss. I attribute a great part of our family's healthy teeth to the floss.

4. Get rid of tartar in the mouth not only by brushing the teeth but the tongue as well. Use your toothbrush or the inverted bowl of a teaspoon. The Yogis do this regularly.

5. A natural mouthwash consists of rose water mixed with your own ratio of plain water.

6. Charcoal or ashes combined with salt have been used for thousands of years to WHITEN teeth. It works!

7. Vitamin A is essential to the development of bones and of tooth enamel. It, and the B-Vitamin, niacin, help to fight gum infections. Vitamin B-6 (always taken with a B-complex tablet) is very effective for tooth decay.

8. A blood-pink toothbrush means that you are in trouble. You may have a deficiency of Vitamin C, which is essential for strong teeth and for healing wounds after an extraction. The vitamin C has been used for scurvy for a long time, but it has been found that the aged are still appallingly deficient of this vitamin.

9. The need for calcium to prevent tooth decay speaks for itself, but Vitamin D is the all-important catalyst of calcium and therefore, the whole calcium family (phosphorus, iodine and phosphates) should be taken as well.

10. Put your foot up on the bathroom sink and straighten the knee, every time you brush your teeth. Not only does it work wonders for your thighs, it keeps you brushing longer, as well.

11. If you cannot brush, at least rinse well after every meal.

Carbohydrates

Carbohydrates are our main source of energy. They are the sugars and starches in our diet. Although the main sources of carbohydrates are breads, cereals, grains, legumes, vegetables and fruit, natural sugars are also found in such diverse foods as meat, cottage cheese, milk and sauerkraut. In fact, you can get all the sugar you need in a day of normal eating without ever touching a grain of refined sugar. The natural sugars can be divided into three distinct groups: simple, double and multiple. Of these, the simple sugars as found in honey, in fruit, especially grapes, and in vegetables such as new Irish potatoes, sweet potatoes, onions, young corn and carrots are absorbed easily. Double sugars, as found in refined sugars, in sprouting seeds and in milk sugar, and multiple sugars as in breads, cereals, rice, peas and legumes, require the process of digestion and take longer to be absorbed. Most of us eat too many carbohydrate foods. They can cause an alkaline mineral deficiency to the detriment of our blood, teeth and bones; they are often responsible for inflammation diseases of the stomach and intestine; they cause a B-vitamin deficiency; they are stored as fat in the belly, the buttocks, the midriff, the double chin; they keep you from eating good nutritious food by satisfying your hunger falsely. It has been found that sedentary people, and those who have a delicate stomach (see Day 11 for digestion) need very little starch, whereas physically active people with a good digestion can tolerate much more. The first should stick to the foods with simple sugars. Test yourself in this way: if you feel sleepy or heavy after a meal in which you have eaten starch, try to cut down on carbohydrate intake. At any rate, learn to make a better choice of carbohydrates. For instance, the potato is the least starchy of the starch foods.

Starch foods

People seem to think that only refined sugars and starches (such as white flour) are considered carbohydrates. You know differently now, but you should be able to understand why these processed "starvation" foods are harmful to you. Many a housewife suffers from hypoglycemia, or low bloodsugar (glucose). Since she may be eating up to 125 pounds of sugar a year from such hidden

63

sources as canned foods, cakes (up to 14 tsp. of sugar in one serving), soft drinks, and even ketchup, the problem is obviously not caused by a lack of sugar. What happens is this: the brain receives the message that food (in the form of carbohydrates) has been received, although it does not yet know that this is usually deficient, refined, poor quality food. Therefore, it signals the pancreas to release insulin to cope with the sudden influx of sugar, a substance which, unlike protein and fats, is assimilated by the body almost immediately. The hunger pangs are now satisfied, but hundreds of cells are actually dying of malnutrition. Insulin, as any diabetic knows, controls the amount of sugar in your blood. If the blood sugar level is low, the liver and the muscles are called upon to release their store of a converted sugar called glycogen; if it is high, the sugar is withdrawn by an injection of more insulin. Concentrated sugar, whether from the teaspoon, a candy-bar, a piece of pie, jam or a soft drink, floods the blood with glucose which causes *extra* insulin to be produced to burn the sugar. This results in too much sugar being removed, which leaves you feeling dizzy, tired, irritable and weak. And since your brain and nervous system can only burn sugar, the lack of it, caused by an over-stimulated pancreas releasing too much insulin, often produces neurotic or psychotic symptoms of depression, anxiety, fatigue, etc. Whereas, had you received your sugar slowly from such foods as meats, milk, fruits (an orange is 10% sugar, a banana 20%), or vegetables (a sweet potato or cooked brown rice is 15%), or unsaturated fats, the digestive process would have introduced the sugar into your system gradually, and you would have received health-sustaining proteins, vitamins and minerals at the same time. A cup of coffee and a doughnut or chocolate bar, then, are the worst food you could eat when you feel low in energy. They bring the blood-sugar level up for an hour without "feeding" you. The slower-acting sugars in proteins, fruits and vegetables, on the other hand, give you a feeling of well-being and energy for five or six hours.

KAREEN'S NUTRITIOUS WEIGHT LOSS DIET

MENU FOR DAY 7

Breakfast
8 oz. orange juice
½ cup whole grain cereal, cooked (wheat or oatmeal) with 2 oz. whole milk
1 tbsp. raw wheat germ and
1 tsp. honey or molasses.

Mid-morning
1 cup 2% milk

Lunch
1 cup alfalfa sprouts
or ¼ head lettuce sprinkled with chopped
parsley
2 tsp. French dressing
6 small canned sardines, well-drained
or 1 broiled filet of sole
1 buttered rye crisp

Mid-afternoon
1 medium apple
or 1" square Cheddar cheese

Dinner
1 cup raw spinach mixed with
½ cup fresh pineapple cubes, garnished with a
couple of onion rings and radish slices
or 1½ cups sauerkraut with apples and onions
½ tbsp. mayonnaise dressing
½ slice baked ham
2 wheat thin crackers

Bedtime snack
1 cup beet borscht*
1 rye crisp

* see recipe section

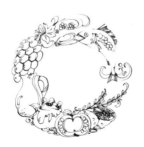

65

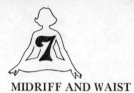

MIDRIFF AND WAIST

Today's breathing exercise is **The Alternate Nostril Breath II** to calm the whole nervous system and purify the bloodstream and relieve insomnia.

1. Sit in a comfortable cross-legged position, back straight.
2. Raise your RIGHT hand and place your RIGHT thumb against your RIGHT nostril, closing it off.
3. Inhale deeply and slowly through the LEFT nostril to the count of four or as long as you can.
4. Close off the LEFT nostril with your ringfinger and retain the breath for a count of 1 - 4 seconds.
5. Open the RIGHT nostril and exhale to the count of four to eight seconds. The longer you can make the exhalation the better. Concentrate on completely emptying the lungs.
6. Repeat steps 3 to 5, three or four times.
7. Reverse the process by inhaling in the RIGHT nostril and exhaling through the LEFT one.
8. Repeat the reverse process three or four times.

The Ear to Knee Pose — reduces the weight in the waist as it relieves backache, tones abdominal muscles, and aids digestion and elimination.

Technique:

1. Sit, legs outstretched and two feet apart.
2. Bend the left leg and bring the foot against the right thigh, letting the knee fall to the side. (Figure 58)
3. Place the right lower arm, palm up, on the right thigh.
4. Turn your body to the left so that it is at right angles with the right leg.
5. Lift your left arm at the side and bring it slowly over your head, elbow straight. (Figure 59)
6. At the same time EXHALE and bend your body to the right, sliding the right arm to the floor on the inside of the leg and forward towards the foot.

7. Grasp the arch of the inside of the right foot with the right
    hand and reach over your head holding the same foot around
    the outside with the left hand. The face will be pointing to
    the front, the ear placed against the knee. (Figure 60)
8. Hold this pose, the left arm over the left ear, for 5 - 20
    seconds, the breath fast and shallow.
9. INHALE, slowly straighten the body, and relax. Repeat on
    the other side.

Do's and Don'ts:

DO make sure that the knee is straight.
DO twist your body to the left for perfect execution of the pose
    and those extra benefits.
DO remember to keep the palm up throughout.

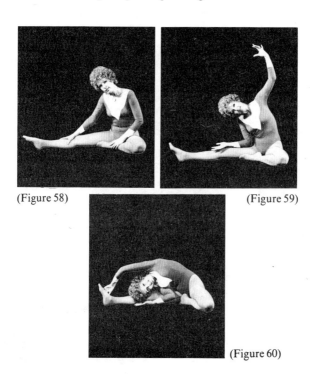

(Figure 58)   (Figure 59)

(Figure 60)

67

The Sideways Swing — reduces the waist line and firms the midriff.

Technique:

1. Sit with legs outstretched.
2. Bend knees and bring feet to the right side. (Figure 61)
3. Inhale, raise both arms over your head and interlace the fingers. (Figure 62)
4. Exhale, bend at the waist, swinging the top of the body to the right as far as it will go. (Figure 63)
5. Hold to a count of 4 or longer. Relax.
6. Repeat three times.
7. Return to the starting position.
8. Bend knees and bring feet to the left side.
9. Repeat steps 3 to 6.

Do's and Don'ts:

DO NOT bend body forward or backward, stay as upright as possible.

(Figure 62)

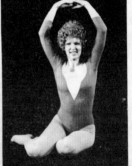

(Figure 61)

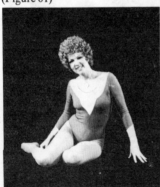

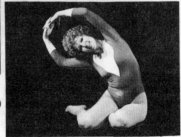

(Figure 63)

68

The Twist — tones and firms the whole body, massages the abdominal organs and twists the spine spirally.

Technique:

1. Sit on the floor, legs outstretched.
2. Spread your legs and bring the RIGHT FOOT against the LEFT THIGH. Press the side of the right knee against the floor. (Figure 64)
3. Bend your left knee and, leaving it sticking up in the air, bring the left foot over the RIGHT KNEE.
4. Set the sole of the LEFT FOOT squarely on the floor. The further back you can bring the foot, the better.
5. Using both hands for support, shift your weight well forward onto the pelvis, to prevent tipping.
6. Raise both your arms and bring them between your chest and the left knee. (Figure 65)
7. Bend your body forward so that your RIGHT SHOULDER is resting against the LEFT KNEE (rather than just the elbow).
8. Now make a fist of your RIGHT HAND and move your RIGHT ARM poker-straight over the RIGHT KNEE that is lying on the floor.
9. Attempt to get hold of the ankle of the left leg. As a beginner, that is nearly impossible, so it is perfectly alright to grasp the right knee.
10. Exhale, levering yourself against the LEFT LEG with the RIGHT arm, now twist to the left.
11. Bend your left arm and bring the back of the hand against the small of the back.
12. Turn your head to the left and look as far left as you can. (Figure 66)
13. Hold this position for 10 - 30 seconds.
14. Slowly unwind.
15. Repeat on the other side.
16. *Variation:* Simple Twist: (Figure 67).

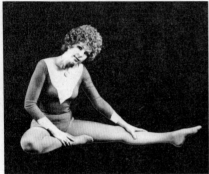

(Figure 64)

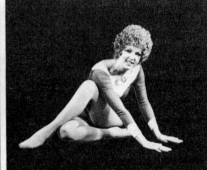

(Figure 65)

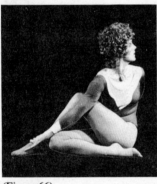

(Figure 66)

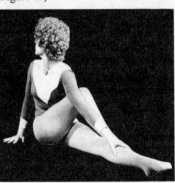

(Figure 67)

Do's and Don'ts:

DO sit well forward on your pelvis.

DO NOT bend your arms as you draw it across the knee.

DO swivel your shoulder or upper arm against the knee to permit
   you to bring your arm around further.

DO remember: if it's the RIGHT knee up, bring both arms to the
   RIGHT and then twist the body to the RIGHT.

Three other poses that reduce the waistline are:
Toe Twist (Day 13, page 124)
Hip Bend (Day 10, page 95)
Pelvic Stretch (Day 9, page 87)

CHANTING THE OM

One of the five meditational forms of yoga is Mantra Yoga. A Mantra is a mystical syllable which is chanted out loud or repeated over and over mentally. The purpose of this repetition is to achieve inner communion by thus learning to concentrate the mind. The Yogis believe that all objects are affected by the vibrations of sound. This is not such a strange thought when one considers that a century ago we would not have believed possible the workings of a wireless radio. By far the most positive and important of all sounds is the mystic syllable OM. It is a word of power. It is generally thought to be one of the names of God and source of all vibration in the Cosmos. The OM, spelled A-U-M in Sanskrit, is a symbol, through its three letters, of everything that is past, present and future. It stands for the three states of experience of Man: waking, dreaming and deep sleep. It represents not only the material, the spiritual and the philosophical spheres but also the vast unknown, a world beyond our comprehension. OM is the most natural sound in the world, even a mute can say it. You can hear it in the BOM of a bell, the AMEN of our prayers, the "oh!" we use to express so many of our feelings. The Yogis believe it to be the basis of all sound. OM is often chanted before a meditation, or on its own. Its vibrations are said to be beneficial to the health by purifying the body and by disciplining the mind. Chanting the OM is a means of elevating the mind on a level above your daily, pedestrian life; it helps the mind to become exalted, to learn to soar.

Practice a few breathing exercises. Now begin to hum the OM. INHALE and start to make the A sound way back in the throat. Slowly change over to the U, finally lingering over a long M sound, with your lips barely touching, all in one long EXHALA-TION. Once you have mastered this technique, meditate on a different thought, such as: "God is light," or "I am immortal" each time you sound the OM. The OM is said to be the source of all light and knowledge.

Day 8

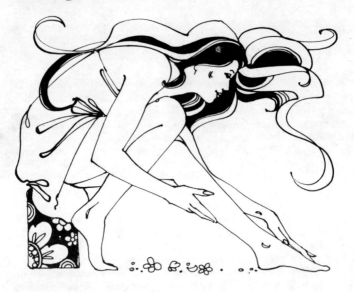

SKIN TONE – STRETCHMARKS, SCARS

What You Should Know!

— The average person's skin covers an area of approximately 2 square meters. (19 sq. ft.)
— The skin, a living and breathing organ, is made up of billions of cells which are constantly being replaced.
— One of this organ's functions is to protect the body from germs and injury, another to regulate heat and the most important is to act as an eliminative organ. When all goes well, the skin becomes an object of beauty, and smooth as alabaster.
— If a vitamin A deficiency exists, the cells that die in the lowest of the four layers of the skin, start to plug the oil sacs and pores and prevent natural oils from reaching the surface. These pores look like constant goose pimples and the skin, due to lack of oils, becomes dry and itchy. The bumps are most common on the back of the arms, the buttocks, side of the hips, the elbows and the knees.
— When no deficiencies exist, the skin has a healthy elasticity. This skintone becomes especially important during pregnancy.

What You Can Do!

1. Every nutrient helps to maintain body elasticity but adequate protein (see list at back — it need not be animal protein) and Vitamin C are most important.
2. Protein can prevent stretchmarks, but care must also be taken not to let the body become water-logged (See Day 14 for Water Retention).
3. Generously applying Vitamin E or coconut oil prevents scarring of tissue. Vitamin E taken internally helps with an easier delivery through increasing muscle elasticity.
4. Cleanse the skin every night to let it breathe. End the bath or shower with a cool rinse for better circulation. Return the acid mantle to the skin with an apple cider vinegar splash in the rinse water. Vegetable oils restore softness to skin.
5. Work on your skintone by taking 10 to 15 minutes to stretch sensuously, sinuously, enjoying every moment of it. MOST IMPORTANT for relaxation is the groaning and moaning, grunting and loud yawning while stretching. Start from a standing position and work your way slowly to a kneeling, then sitting, finally lying position. Stretch all the while; your skin reflects your inner state of mind.
6. To plump up tissue, dissolve lecithin granules in warm water then add cold pressed vegetable oils and rub into the skin for an all day beauty treatment.

Vitamins & Minerals

Physically, we are what we eat. Mentally, we are what we think. But if we don't eat properly, we can't think properly. We may become irritable, depressed, anxious or merely fatigued. It has long been known that food has great powers over our energy and health, but it took modern science to divide food into four main sections: vitamins, minerals, proteins, and essential fatty acids. Of these, the first two play an important and interlocking role. Without the preparatory body-building work done by the minerals, the vitamins could not work nearly so well. For a superior, healthy and energetic family, you must have an adequate supply of the four main food groups. However this is very difficult in this age, because of the interference we have run with nature. Now, because of chemical fertilizers and insecticides (which upset

the natural balance inherent in soil), because of the refining process of foods, and because of chemical additives in our foods to permit longer shelf-life (which largely benefits the supplier rather than the customer) a carrot is no longer a carrot. For how high a vitamin A (carotene) content this vegetable has is entirely dependent on the soil in which it grew and on the way in which it was stored.

Every housewife should know that vitamins are either fat-soluble (A, D, E and K) or water-soluble (B and C). Water-solubility explains the saying "throw out the vegetables and keep the vegetable water". (Whenever possible, cook with a French steamer, so that the produce is never in contact with the water. Make soups from the cooking water and from canned vegetable liquids.) Some vitamins are destroyed by light (B^2), others by air (Vit. A and Vit. C, when heated), by heat, by pasteurization (B^1), by chlorine (Vit. E), by alkalies or by cooking. For example, when making your own yogurt, you should always cover the container with a cloth to protect the B^2 from light.

The carrot I mentioned earlier is excellent as concerns roughage and teeth-exercising properties, but for deriving Vitamin A, this tough root-vegetable needs to be softened by par-boiling or juicing. A carrot also contains four very important minerals: iodine, zinc, copper and iron. Minute amounts of the first are very necessary, but iron and calcium are the most common mineral deficiencies in North America, according to the recent Nutrition Canada Survey. This, surprisingly, was not just true of women, but also of teenagers and of men who had bleeding ulcers. Iron plays a large part in delivering oxygen to the cells, to keep you from becoming anaemic and contributes to a healthy, rosy complexion. Calcium, always in conjunction with magnesium, is an excellent nerve relaxer and the need for it is increased before menstruation and before puberty. All mothers know that it is needed for bone and tooth formation. Scientists now suspect that minerals, especially trace minerals, are even more important than vitamins. There is no doubt that most North Americans are severely deficient in the B-vitamins (brewer's yeast, molasses, yogurt, wheat germ, liver, organ meats, grains and legumes), which spell ENERGY, RESISTANCE TO INFECTION and STRESS, GOOD DIGESTION and LONGEVITY. (See chart for deficiency symptoms).

74

In the back of the book we have a Vitamin and Mineral chart to guide you in your choice of foods. Decide if you have a deficiency and then try to supplement your diet with the foods which are rich in the lacking nutrient. If this seems inadequate, you may have to resort to supplementing with vitamin and mineral tablets derived from NATURAL sources.

KAREEN'S NUTRITIOUS WEIGHT LOSS DIET

MENU FOR DAY 8

Breakfast	½ cup plain yogurt with ½ cup fresh or unsweetened frozen strawberries 1 wheat germ or soy muffin + ½ pat butter **or** 1 slice pumpernickel with ½ pat butter 1 tbsp. honey.
Mid-morning	2 tsp. flaked yeast **or** 1 tsp. soy flour Mixed in 1 cup orange juice
Lunch	¾ cup raw grated cabbage ½ cup raw grated beets 1 grated medium carrot 1 chopped green onion with 1 tbsp. safflower oil & apple cider vinegar 1 buttered rye crisp
Mid-afternoon	6 apricot halves (dried) **or** ½ cantaloupe
Dinner	125 gr. (4 oz.) broiled beef liver or one chicken breast **or** 1 cup spinach 1 medium steamed onion
Bedtime snack	1 medium apple **or** 1 cup fresh pineapple **or** ½ banana with 1 tbsp. coconut

ABDOMEN

Today's breathing exercise is **The Digestive Cycle** for better digestion.

1. Sit, comfortably cross-legged, hands on knees.
2. Now describe a circle with your upper body in a clockwise movement, by
3. Leaning back exhaling, and pulling the abdomen IN, then
4. Bending forward inhaling and pushing the abdomen OUT.
5. Repeat 4 times, then perform the same movement in an anti-clockwise direction. The rhythm is: lean backward — exhale — pull tummy IN — bend forward — inhale — push tummy OUT.

The Bow — tones and firms the muscles of the abdomen, arms, legs and back. It reduces weight in the hips and buttocks.

Technique:

1. Lie face down on your abdomen, hands by your side.
2. Bend your knees and bring them close to your buttocks.
3. INHALE and grasp your legs at the ankles, one at a time. (Figure 68)
4. Now EXHALE and lift your knees off the floor by pulling the ankles *away* from the hands. You will still be tightly holding on, but it is the *away* motion rather than a *down* pull that will do the trick.
5. Lift your head at the same time. (Figure 69)
6. Hold the position for 5 - 10 seconds at the first, increasing to 30 seconds at 5 seconds a week. Breathe normally.
7. Slowly relax and rest for a while.
8. Repeat twice more.

Do's and Don'ts:

DO come out of the exercise slowly.

DO pull the ankles "up and away" rather than down, to get those stubborn knees off the ground.

DON'T collapse in a heap. You will get more exercise for your time.

DON'T be alarmed if the body rocks a little with the breathing motions. It has a beneficial massaging effect.

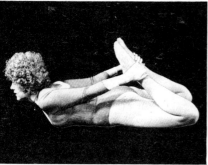

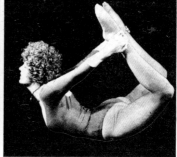

| (Figure 68) | (Figure 69) |

The Sideleg Lift — firms the hips and tightens the tummy. It's really as good as doing two exercises.

Technique:

1. Sit, with the legs extended.
2. Lean back and place the hands straight down from the shoulder, the fingers pointing to the sides.
3. Bend your elbows slightly and raise the toes no more than 3 inches off the floor. (Figure 70)
4. Now move the legs slowly over the floor to the RIGHT without raising them. Go as far as you can, rolling over the RIGHT hip.
5. Exhale, lift the legs as far as they will go, shifting your weight slightly to the LEFT, so that the right arm is straightened. The left one stays bent. Hold 3 - 4 seconds or as long as possible. (Figure 71)
6. Bring the legs down ON THE SIDE, rolling again over the hip and only then bring them forward slowly, the feet only 3 inches off the floor. (Figure 72)
7. Repeat on the other side. As you improve, try going from one side to the other without stopping in the middle.

Do's and Don'ts:

DON'T lean too far back while performing this exercise.
DO straighten the RIGHT arm when the legs are up on the RIGHT.
DON'T raise the legs higher than 3 inches while moving them over
the floor.
DO come down all the way over on the side, not towards the front.

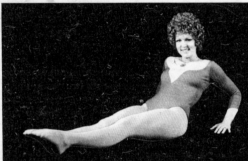

(Figure 70)

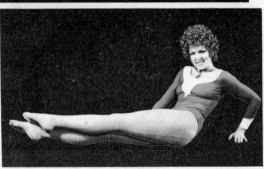

(Figure 71)

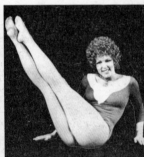

(Figure 72)

The Sit-Up — strengthens the back, tightens the derriere and firms
and flattens the abdominal muscles.

Technique:

1. Lie on your back, knees bent *just* enough so that the whole
    foot is touching the floor. (No further)
2. Place your hands on the thighs. (Figure 73)

78

3. Lift your head slowly and raise your upper body to a 30° angle off the floor, sliding the hands up the legs. Depending on the length of your arms, the fingertips should barely be touching the bent knee-cap.
4. Keeping your back as straight as possible, hold the position 5 - 30 seconds. (Figure 74)
5. Slowly lower your trunk. Relax.
6. Repeat 3 - 5 times more.
7. *Variation:* Put hands behind the head and do 5 slow sit-ups. (Figure 75)

Do's and Don'ts:

DO NOT go much further than a 30° angle. If the exercise comes too easily, if the rectal muscles of the abdomen are not standing out in a taut ridge, you may be sure that you have gone too far. Ease back a little.

DO breathe normally.

Three other poses that help to firm the tummy muscles are:
The Crow (Day 6, page 58)
Ear to Knee Pose (Day 7, page 66)
Rock 'n Rolls (Day 14, page 132)

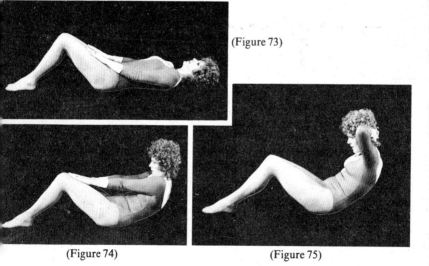

(Figure 73)

(Figure 74)   (Figure 75)

MEDITATING THROUGH VISUALIZATION

Sit comfortably, your back straight, your head supported. Take a deep breath. With your eyes closed and your hands quietly folded in your lap, imagine yourself standing at the top of the highest building in the whole world — a brand new skyscraper. It is so high that as you stand there at the railing, you feel as though your head is touching the sky. Look all around you. Imagine a breath-taking view. Look far away, over the city into the country. Admire the towering mountains capped with snow; follow the path of a river winding sinuously through green hills and meadows; let your eyes wander over the patchwork quilt of color. Drink in the view. It is food and drink to the soul — soothing and balming. Make it a part of you.

Go now into the building and up to the elevator. The building is brand new; no one has been there before you. As the door opens you step into a most pleasant little room. The wood-panelled elevator is warm and inviting, with soft lights and gentle background music. Your feet touch the thick pile of orange-brown carpet, deep, and luxurious. The doors close quietly behind you. Push the downward button. With hardly a sense of wonder, you soon realize that the elevator is very, very slow. You don't mind; it gives you a chance to relax and rest awhile. Lie down. Curl into the deep, soft pile of the carpet. Its new and pleasant smell envelopes you. The orange fibres, the golden light, the cozy warmth make you feel so peaceful, as you sink down. The carpet receives you, you become one with it, you give yourself into it. The elevator is slowly moving down, down, down; on and on, forever and ever. Let yourself go with it, float down, down, down. With a slight smile on your lips, give yourself up to the warmth, the peace, the serenity. Think only of positive things. Transcend the worldly worries, leave them behind you. Sink down: light, weightless, happy. No thoughts. Smoothly down, down, down. Lighter and lighter, floating, peaceful, silent.

Day 9

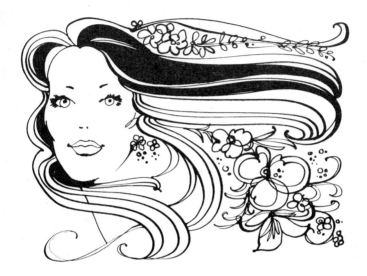

HAIR – CARE AND EXERCISE

What You Should Know!

— If you wanted your hair as shiny and glistening as a mink's pelt,
you would have to eat a diet consisting of fresh liver, fish, tripe,
lungs, raw red meat, prepared cereal of whole grains, tomato
puree, skim milk powder, wheat germ meal and vitamin and
mineral supplements.
— Each and every one of your hairs has its own little factory – the
matrix – a cluster of cells from which the hair grows.
— Leading to the root of the hair are tiny arteries which bring
rich, freshly oxygenated blood, if your diet has been good.
— Nearer to the scalp lie the sebaceous glands, whose function it
is to lubricate the hair and skin. This is why brushing has always
been a beauty treatment. It distributes the oils along the hair to
the tips and cleanses it at the same time.

81

What You Can Do!

1. Cut down on all junk foods, particularly sugar and white flour starches, and soft drinks.
2. Eat a diet with adequate protein (vegetable or animal) which can also be taken in the form of brewer's yeast, a *must* vitamin for hair.
3. Supplement with minerals such as potassium, zinc, copper, iodine, phosphorus and sulphur in your food.
4. Eat a diet rich in viable seeds (those capable of sprouting) and sprouts: germinating seeds for sprouting hair!
5. Cod-liver oil, or pure vegetable oil, especially wheat germ oil, are recommended for healthy, bouncing, shiny hair.
6. Raw grains, seeds and nuts help production of enzymes, hormones, vitamins and minerals for healthy hair.
7. Increase the circulation to the scalp by massage, the use of a slantboard, or the head- and shoulderstand.
8. A good waveset after a shampoo is beer or skim milk. If your hair is excessively oily use 1 tbsp. of salt added to the skim milk.
9. Brush your hair, with a natural bristle brush only up to 100 times, (only 25 if you have very oily hair).
10. Give yourself a protein treatment: egg yolk or mayonnaise left on the hair for half an hour.
11. Use shampoo with a natural PH factor or one rich in lanolin. Follow it with an apple cider vinegar or lemon rinse for squeaky cleanliness and a correct acid balance.
12. Make an "instant" shampoo for oily hair, by beating up egg whites and distributing them over the head; let dry, brush out.
13. If your hair is dry, give it a 15 minute castor oil or vegetable oil treatment just before the shampoo.
14. Always have a regular trim — it will help your hair to grow.
15. Do not stretch the hair through tight hairdos, rough brushing or sleeping on curlers. Look in the list at the end of the book for nutrients, in the form of food, which are good for your hair.

Fats and Proteins

The importance of an adequate supply of proteins in your diet is obvious. Protein is the stuff of which most of you is made, from the protoplasm of your cells to the skin which covers you. If you are deficient in protein you develop symptoms of anemia (pallor, fatigue), swollen ankles at night and puffy eyes, face and hands in the morning, loss of muscle tone, and wrinkles. However, if you suffer from foul gases, constipation and fatigue, you may well be eating too much protein. Contrary to what you may have heard, animal protein is not absolutely necessary or better for you than vegetable protein. Often, meat-eating brings with it disease. Vegetarians, for example, are usually free of arthritis. People who live very long have been moderate in their habits all of their lives and usually have eaten meat only two or three times a year. (Some work being done with cancer in Sweden and the U.S. suggests that over-indulgence of protein may be a factor in the disease). Protein is essential for new cell growth, for cell repair and for the structural make-up of the cell. But for food digestion, protein must be properly combined with other foods. (See Day 11, page 101). Protein is a more complex substance than fats or carbohydrates. Good, easily-digested sources are milk, eggs, nuts, soybeans and the protein of green, leafy vegetables, says Dr. Alice Chase in her book NUTRITION FOR HEALTH.

Briefly, the body needs approximately 32 different amino acids. Of these, it can manufacture all but eight essential amino acids, which we call, when they are *all* present in one meal, a Complete Protein. This is what happens. When food enters the mouth, the chemicals in the saliva start to break down starches. But, gross protein foods are attacked by enzymes (also a group of small proteins) and broken down into smaller portions called amino acids in the stomach. Meats contain all eight essential amino acids. However a complete protein can also be produced by proper food combining of other food sources. A surprising list of proteins: meat, cheese, milk, avocados, nuts, soybeans, all cereals, dry beans, dry peas, peanuts, olives, brewer's yeast (flaked), wheatgerm, soybean flour, non-instant powdered milk, cottonseed. Proteins are not, surprisingly, our most concentrated form of energy. This claim belongs to the fats and oils.

The fatty acids in oils are divided into two groups: saturated and unsaturated. Our body needs only the latter. Products such as butter, lard, pasteurized milk, cream, meat and poultry fats,

contain both kinds of fats. Vegetable oils become saturated through hydrogenation, a process which solidifies the oil and thereby robs fat-soluble vitamins of their protection on their journey through the digestive tract. Experts say that this raises the cholesterol level and they reject lard, margarine, solid cooking fats, processed cheeses and *hydrogenated* peanut butter as contributing causes to gall-stone formation, heart disease and strokes. For example, an egg fried in butter appreciably raises its cholesterol count, whereas one fried in oil does not raise the cholesterol level at all. Paradoxically, oil has the power of keeping the complexion clear and smooth; it helps to lose weight because it releases water from the cells, because "fat eats fat", because sugar is changed to fat more rapidly if essential fatty acids are under-supplied; and it keeps the blood cholesterol level down. A combination of adequate, good-source protein and oil is an unbeatable source of energy.

KAREEN'S NUTRITIOUS WEIGHT LOSS DIET

MENU FOR DAY 9

Breakfast	6 dried apricot halves
	1 cup cooked oatmeal porridge
	with ½ cup 2% milk
Mid-morning	8 almonds and
	1 tbsp. sunflower seeds
	or 1 cup alfalfa sprouts
Lunch	2 poached eggs
	1 slice light rye toast with 1 pat butter
	or 1 muffin (soy or wheat germ)
	with ½ pat butter
Mid-afternoon	1 cup celery and carrot sticks
	with tomato, sliced
Dinner	4 oz. steamed salmon or cod or halibut
	1 cup steamed broccoli
	1 cup steamed carrots
Bedtime snack	1 apple
	or ½ cantaloupe

BUTTOCKS

Today's Breathing exercise is **The Alternate Nostril Breath III** to aerate the lungs, refresh the body, free the mind of any depressed feelings, and combat insomnia.

1. Sit in a comfortable cross-legged position, back straight.
2. Raise your RIGHT hand and place your thumb against your RIGHT nostril, closing it off.
3. Inhale deeply and slowly through the LEFT nostril to the count of four.
4. Close off the LEFT nostril with your ringfinger and retain the breath for a count of 1 to 4 seconds.
5. Open the RIGHT nostril and exhale to the count of 4 to 8 seconds. The longer you can make the exhalation, the better. Concentrate on completely emptying the lungs.
6. Breathe in through that same RIGHT nostril to the count of 4.
7. Close off the nostril with the ringfinger again and hold to the count of 1 to 4 seconds.
8. Exhale through the LEFT nostril to the count of 4 to 8 seconds. This makes up one round.
9. Repeat these rounds of alternate nostril breathing five more times, or up to ten minutes if you are concerned about insomnia.
10. Practise a ratio of 4:4:8, if at all possible.

Today's other exercises that are excellent for firming buttocks, hips and thighs are:

Bow (Day 8, page 76)
Cobra (Day 6, page 59)
Sit-Up (Day 8, page 78)

The Half-Locust — strengthens and firms the buttocks, abdomen and thighs and helps to reduce weight in these areas.

Technique:

1. Lie on your stomach, hands by your sides, palms up.
2. Raise your head and bring the front of the chin against the floor. (Figure 76)
3. Pressing the arms against the floor, INHALE and slowly raise the right leg straight up in the back as far as you can. Keep the left leg straight. (Figure 77)

4. Hold the breath and the pose from 5 - 10 seconds, EXHALE, slowly lowering the leg. Relax.
5. Repeat on the other side, making sure that the body weight is not rolled to the side of the out-stretched leg.
6. As a variation, make fists, thumbs extended, index finger side of the fist down, and place them under your body between the hips.
7. Another variation is to clasp your hands with crossed wrists, arms straight under the abdomen. (Figure 78)

Do's and Don'ts:

DO practise the **Half-Locust** only, for several weeks, to strengthen a weak back.

DO use the excellent leverage of pressing your chin and your arms firmly against the floor.

DO try to make your knees as straight as possible.

DO come out of the pose slowly. You nullify a great deal of your effort by collapsing.

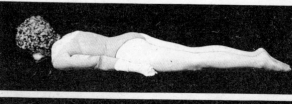

(Figure 76)

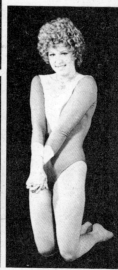

(Figure 77)

(Figure 78)

The Pelvic Stretch — strengthens and firms the legs and hips as well as the thighs and abdomen.

Technique:

1. Kneel, resting on the heels, legs together.
2. Place your right hand on the floor behind you, elbow straight, fingers pointing back.
3. Place the left hand on the other side, having both hands straight down from the shoulders.
4. Let your head hang back. (Figure 79)
5. Push up on the pelvis as far as it will go and hold for 5 - 30 seconds. (Figure 80)
6. Slowly lower yourself back onto your heels and come forward into the **Curling Leaf**, head resting on the floor, chest against the knees, buttocks resting on the heels, arms resting by your side. This helps to offset the extended backward bend.
7. Repeat steps 1 - 5, angling your hands further back each time. (Figure 81) Always return to the **Curling Leaf**.
8. Perform three times.

Do's and Don'ts:

DO NOT forget to push your pelvis up, so that the buttocks are no longer resting on the heels. The whole front of your body should describe an arch.

DO bring the body forward after each pose to off-set the extreme backward stretch.

(Figure 79)

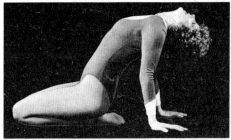

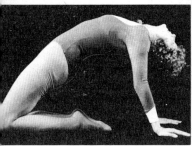

(Figure 80)

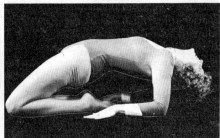

(Figure 81)

9

The Reverse Arch — relieves backache as it firms the hips and buttocks.

Technique:

1. Lie on your back, knees bent, feet flat on the floor, arms by your side.
2. Pull the feet as close to the buttocks as possible, without straining. (Figure 82)
3. Exhale and slowly tilt the pelvis up, pushing the small of the back (the hollow) against the floor. The pelvis is NOT lifted, only tilted. (Figure 83)
4. Hold the pose, exhale and lower the pelvis. Repeat once more.
5. Now, inhale and slowly push the buttocks and lower body up as high as you can. (Figure 84)
6. Shift the weight towards the shoulders, relax the arms, and breathe normally.
7. Hold 5 - 30 seconds. Exhale and relax slowly, bringing the back down vertebra by vertebra. Repeat three to four times.

Do's and Don'ts:

DO only tilt the pelvis without lifting it, in steps 1 - 4. The buttocks should not be wholly off the floor. The feeling should almost be one of pinching the buttocks together.

DON'T keep the weight on the arms. Shift the weight to the shoulders and relax the arms as much as possible.

DO enjoy the delightful stretching sensation in your upper legs.

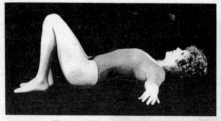

(Figure 82)

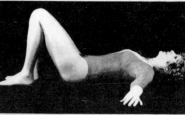

(Figure 83)

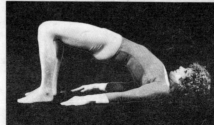

(Figure 84)

88

PRAYING

What is the difference between prayer and meditation? Both are meant to be spiritual experiences, a communing with a higher being, whether He be in heaven or within ourselves. In meditation nothing is asked for, but in prayer we often ask God for things: for a new house, for health, for a lost key, for a new job, instead of asking Him for guidance.

Yet Jesus said: "Take no thought, saying, What shall we eat? or What shall we drink? or Wherewithal shall we be clothed? ... for your heavenly Father knoweth that ye have need of all these things. But seek ye first the Kingdom of God, and his righteousness; and all these things shall be added unto you." If you are seeking peace of mind, whether through meditation or prayer, you must stop wanting and start communing. This is where prayer and meditation can become one, when the mind is brought to rest and the spirit takes over. In writing this, I asked a dear friend to give me her idea of prayer. None is better qualified to answer this question than she. A devout person, she has made a total success of her life. She is charming, cheerful, enthusiastic, positive, much younger looking than her 52 years; she has combined a career in fashion with raising five exceptionally fine sons who neither smoke, drink nor carouse, and who are both athletic and musical. My friend is happily married, but has experienced heartbreak through the death of two children, one, the only daughter. This is what she said: "I always start out thanking the Heavenly Father for our blessings — and we *have* been blessed. Then I ask him to bless this house and to give us the strength to endure our trials; I ask for guidance whenever I am in doubt and for enlightenment to help me find a way out of a problem." But she never, never asks for a specific thing, only light and knowledge. She believes firmly that "God helps those who help themselves." At the end of her prayers she always adds: "Thy will be done."

How much is prayer, how much meditative truth? It's hard to measure, but there can be little doubt that they each can improve the quality of the other.

Day 10

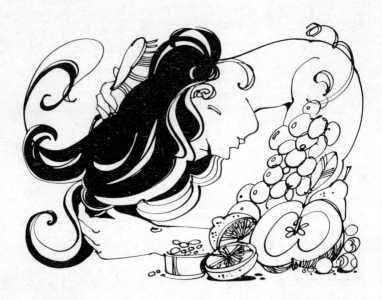

HAIR PROBLEMS AND VITAMINS

What You Should Know!

— There seems to be a definite connection between heavy coffee-drinking and grey, balding hair. A deficiency of the B-vitamins, biotin, inositol, folic acid and pantothenic acid is caused by coffee-drinking. Copper deficiency is also a villain here.

— A lack of the B-vitamins, together with an over-indulgence of large quantities of sweets, starches, animal fats, alcohol, chocolate and cream and butter can cause dandruff. The excessive fat and sugar intake cannot be absorbed by the body and can cause extra secretion of sebum.

— Dandruff flack consists of minute flecks of dead skin, constantly being replaced by new skin, which have glued together in a larger crust. Dandruff, in turn, is one of the causes in falling-out hair. Others are radio-active fallout, heredity, and B Vitamin and other multiple nutritional deficiencies.

What You Can Do!

1. If you have a real problem, go to a dermatologist. After all, you go to a dentist when you have a toothache.
2. Adelle Davis says that a much-neglected Vitamin B is Inositol, which helped experimental animals to grow hair.
3. Lack of Vitamin A can cause dry hair and itching. (See list).
4. The colour of hair cannot be restored by *synthetic* vitamins, but good results can be had temporarily by a diet adequate in natural B vitamins (see Charts).
5. Fresh fruits and vegetables, eaten raw or only partially steamed, provide many of the needed nutrients.
6. Radio-active fallout can be countered by kelp tablets (seaweed is considered a "wonder food"; it beautifies skin and hair, gives energy and acts as an appetite reducer before meals), and vitamins, particularly the B vitamins.
7. *Free* vitamins and minerals are found in sprouts, an excellent factor in growing lots of healthy hair. When seeds are sprouted the Vitamin content increases variously from 10% to 1000%.

Food Combining

Why do animals in their natural state not suffer from ulcers, cancers and tumors of their digestive tract? What can we learn from their behavior? — Simplicity. Animals rarely overeat, but above all, they eat very simply. They never combine carbohydrates or acids with their proteins. Some animals and birds even eat alternate foods on alternate days. Such simplicity of menu results in a minimum of fermentation, putrefaction and forming of poisons. Thus, the digestive catalysts, known as enzymes, can do their all-important work most efficiently. Enzymes — small proteins — are present in every atom and molecule of the cells, plant or animal. They are the source of all energy. Digestive enzymes are very limited and specific as to action. Each group of enzymes acts only upon a specific food group (or sub-groups), and then only at *certain stages of digestion.*

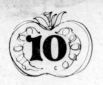

Digestion of starches starts in the mouth with an enzyme called ptyalin, in the saliva. Ptyalin is destroyed by the acid in fruits and vinegar. Therefore, do not eat acids and starches in the same meal. For best digestion, starches need an alkaline medium. Proteins, however, require an acid medium and are digested in the stomach. Protein and starch are not compatible in the same meal. Were you to eat the meat or cheese in your sandwich first and the bread after, or the steak first and the potato after, the stomach could cope with the situation; it would digest the protein in its lower end (distal), and keep the starch in the upper end (quiescent) while a form of salivary digestion is carried on for another two hours. It is the thorough mixing together through chewing and saliva of both types of food at the same time, which causes the trouble. Two *different* proteins should not be taken at the same meal, either. Milk, for instance, says Dr. H.M. Shelton in FOOD COMBINING MADE EASY, has gastric juice poured on it in the last hour of digestion, meat in the first. Eggs receive yet another timing of the juices. You may eat two different kinds of meat together, or two different nuts, but milk should be taken on its own. Also incompatible are: meat plus eggs; meat and nuts; meat plus cheese, cheese and nuts. *A combination of acid and protein is not advisable either* since the stomach-enzyme (pepsin) works only in an acid medium of its own making (hydrochloric acid). Adding acid fruits or vinegar actually prevents the flow of gastric juices, which causes putrefaction. Nuts and cheese, because of their fat content, are permissible with acid fruits since the two have approximately the same timing of gastric juices. Fat, however, has a depressing or inhibiting effect on digestion, which can last several hours; so, *fat and protein should not be combined.* If this is unavoidable, then green, uncooked vegetables with the meal will offset the inhibiting effect of fat. Since they act similarly to fat, sugars must be avoided with either protein or starches. If taken alone, sugar is digested by neither the mouth nor the stomach, but by the small intestine. When eaten with other food, they ferment quickly and cause an acid, sour stomach with burps and indigestion. That means no sugar or jam on cereal or toast. Shelton also recommends that starchy meals (potatoes, bread, baked beans, rice) be eaten at noon and protein meals be eaten at night. Fruits are eaten as a separate meal at breakfast. Rest should follow all meals.

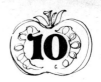

If you want good digestion without putrefaction or fermentation, please follow these rules:

YES

MEAT	+	NON-STARCHY VEGETABLES
CHEESE & NUTS	+	GREEN VEGETABLES
FRUITS	+	NON-STARCHY VEGETABLES
ACIDS	+	NUTS, AVOCADOS and CHEESE (cottage cheese and fruit salad)
STARCH	+	VEGETABLES (preferably non-starchy)
FRUITS	+	ALL KINDS in one fruit meal
VEGETABLES	+	ALL KINDS — IF no protein is in the same meal.
WATER —		ten minutes before the meal, but not during or for three to four hours after the meal.

NO

ACID	+	STARCH (i.e. acidic and sweet fruit in a salad)
ACID	+	PROTEIN (except for cheese, nuts and avocados)
PROTEIN	+	STARCH (except if protein is taken first in the same meal)
PROTEIN	+	PROTEIN (except for meat + meat, nuts + nuts, etc.)
FAT	+	PROTEIN (except with green, uncooked vegetables)
SUGAR	+	PROTEIN
SUGAR	+	STARCH
MILK	+	ANYTHING (except with cod-liver oil)
MELONS	+	ANYTHING (eat them in a meal to themselves)
NUTS	+	SWEET FRUIT (i.e. raisins, bananas, figs, dates)
DESSERTS	+	ANYTHING (try to avoid them)
FRUITS	+	ANYTHING (eat them as a separate meal)
COLD DRINKS	+	ANYTHING (iced drinks at any time are most inhibiting to the digestion)

KAREEN'S NUTRITIOUS WEIGHT LOSS DIET

MENU FOR DAY 10

Breakfast ½ grapefruit
6 dried apricot halves
2 eggs scrambled with milk

Mid-morning 1 medium apple
or 1" square cheddar cheese or muenster or gruyere cheese

Lunch	Pineapple blender drink (with sunflower seeds instead of egg):—
	1 cup pineapple juice
	1 tbsp. non-instant skim milk powder
	or 1 tsp. soy flour
	2 tsp. yeast flakes
	1 tsp. wheat germ (raw)
	½ banana
	2 tsp. hulled sunflower seeds
	(The whole above luncheon may be substituted for the Day 6 Salad)
Mid-afternoon	1 tbsp. honey
	or 2 tsp. cream cheese
	1 rye crisp
Dinner	100 gr. (4 oz) serving parsleyed sole fillets
	or shrimp with lemon juice
	¾ cup mashed potato with 1 pat butter
	raw carrot & celery sticks
Bedtime snack	1 cup beet borscht
	or 1 cup chicken broth with 1 tsp. soyflour.

HIPS

Today's breathing exercise is **Breathing Away Pain** or **Positive Breathing**. To rid your mind of negative thoughts or pain, or simply to give yourself a more positive image of yourself, try this:

1. Lie on your back and breathe deeply and rhythmically.
2. Think positively that you are going to breathe away the pain or negative thought.
3. Inhale, now direct all your life-force, all the energy you derive from every inhalation, to the pain (a headache, a toothache, backache, menstrual pain, etc.)
4. Exhale, concentrate on breathing the pain away with every exhalation.
5. It has been found helpful to drink half a glass of cool water before starting this breathing exercise.

The Hip Bend — provides an excellent stretch on one side as it tightens waist and midriff on the other.

Technique:

1. Stand with feet about one meter apart, (1 yard) with arms clasped overhead. (Figure 85) Inhale.
2. Now exhale and bend the body as far as possible to the LEFT. This is a sideways bend, do not let body bend forward at the waist. Hold for 5 seconds, holding the breath. If you hold longer, breathe normally, bending further with each exhalation. (Figure 86)
3. Repeat to the right.
4. Repeat both sides three more times.

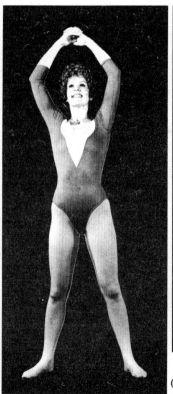

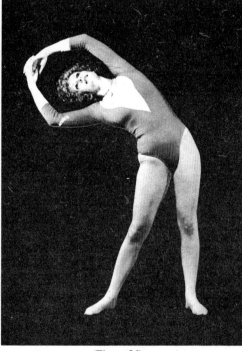

(Figure 86)

(Figure 85)

10

Do's and Don'ts:

DO shift the body weight to the right with the hips if the arms go to the left, and vice versa.

DON'T tense, let yourself go loose with each exhalation.

The Hip Walk — works on the buttocks and hips while you are exercising your arms and legs. A good exercise for young and old.

Technique:

1. Sit with legs outstretched. Keep knees straight throughout.
2. Bend the elbows, bringing the hands loosely forward in front of your chest. (Figure 87)
3. Start walking briskly on your hips pushing forward the heel of one leg first, then the other.
4. Roll over each hip, tilting to the side with each "step" until one buttock is off the floor. (Figure 88)
5. Let the arms walk with you by bringing the RIGHT elbow forward when the LEFT buttock is off the floor, and vice versa.
6. Walk forward to the wall, then back.

Do's and Don'ts:

DO "bump" against the floor vigorously, to massage fatty tissue.
DO push heels forward, rather than toes.

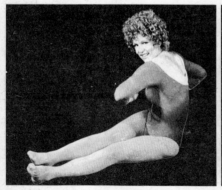

(Figure 87)

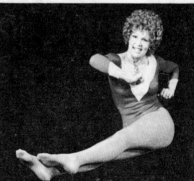

(Figure 88)

The Roll Twist — puts the weight of half your body on the outside hip to help break down the fat cells while the effort firms your abdomen.

Technique:

1. Lie back with both arms outstretched to the sides.
2. INHALE, bend the knees and pull them against the chest. (Figure 89)
3. Now EXHALE and roll the knees to the left, while turning the head to the right. Keep both shoulders on the floor. Hold.
4. INHALE, bring the legs up and repeat the roll over to the right, turning the head to the left, and hold.
5. Repeat the complete sequence at least three more times, with a holding position or in a continuous rhythm roll.
6. *Variation:* Instead of bringing legs to chest, simply pull the heels to the buttocks, feet on the floor, twist. (Figure 90)
7. *Variation:* (which is excellent for waist, midriff and thighs) with legs outstretched, raise one and bring it on the floor over the other one, perpendicular to arms. Turn head the other way. (Figure 91)

Do's and Don'ts:

DON'T go all the way to the floor, if your shoulders tend to come up. Rest knees on a cushion instead.

DO enjoy the gently therapeutic twist to the spine.

(Figure 90)

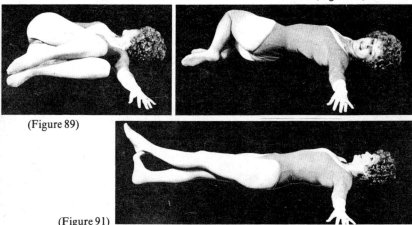

(Figure 89)

(Figure 91)

Other poses that help reduce the fat hips are:
Half-Locust (Day 9, page 86)
Side Leg Lift (Day 8, page 77)
Side Raise (Day 11, page 103)

MEDITATING ON A SENTENCE

We've talked of the need for the modern world to have constant diversion. Our frenetic activities cause a pouring outward of our energies. The result is the loss of ability to concentrate, to think, to make decisions and to solve problems. When we finally become aware of our headlong rush, we feel the need for stillness, for solitude, for truth and knowledge. And this we can find in the practice of concentration.

Picture a beautiful, still pond in the middle of the forest. Not a ripple disturbs its surface — it is smooth as glass. When you bend forward, you can see your own image as clearly as in a mirror. But let a mosquito skim the surface, let a slight breeze spring up, let a fish jump — and your image will be ugly and distorted, out of proportion.

So it is with meditation. When you have cleared your mind of all debris (ripples), when you have concentrated on an object (candle or apple), when you have visualized it, have contemplated on it, have thought about it from all angles; when you have totally exhausted the topic — a stillness sets in. You think: "What next?" That is the time when you will suddenly be inspired. You will think things you have never thought before. You will feel illuminated, inspired, light-filled.

Today we will move one step further from the examination of a concrete object such as the apple and from the repetition of one word, to the repetition and contemplation of a sentence. This can be any thought or sentence you like, according to your philosophy or religion. But let it be positive and inspiring. My own favorite is: "God is light". As I meditate on this sentence (repeating it endlessly in my mind) I visualize the light. I try to visualize the light in the middle of my forehead; I let it spread to my heart, to my entire body, through the room, filling the house, the street, the city, the country, the continent until the whole world is ablaze with the light of love.

Day 11

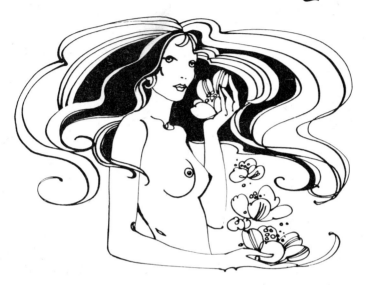

CELLULITE

What You Should Know!

— Four out of five women will eventually suffer from cellulite, whether they are overweight or not. Cellulite is caused by deposits of body fluids, fats and toxins between the muscles and the skin. It is a kind of poison in the connective tissues which the body should have eliminated.
— Contributive factors are poor elimination, poor nutrition, tension, lack of exercise, not enough liquids, hormone changes and, minimally, heredity. Even air pollution and improper breathing may be factors.
— The test is to squeeze together, between thumb and middle finger, a patch of skin. If the skin looks dimpled and rippled like a big orange rind, you may be plagued by cellulite.
— It usually appears in the thighs, hips, buttocks, abdomen and the inside of the knees. Women fear it for the way it makes them look in a bathing suit.
— Since cellulite is a relatively new problem to physicians, they do not agree on how to treat it. Some work is being done on it in Europe. Exercise is important, and so is gently kneading,

stroking massage. Yoga is invaluable here, with its breathing and relaxation exercises recommended in the fight to rid the body of poisons.

What You Can Do!

1. Vitamin C helps to form and maintain the strong, cement-like stiff-jellied collagen known as connective tissue which holds together all the cells of the body. Before this jelly can set, adequate calcium must be present. Then the connective tissue is strong enough to ward off viruses, poisons, and dangerous drugs.
2. Vitamin C often combines with toxic substances and the two are then excreted together.
3. Trace minerals are also very important in ridding the body of toxins, especially copper, zinc, sodium and potassium.
4. Recommended in the battle against cellulite are brewer's yeast, iodine and plenty of raw salads and vegetables for roughage. You will win the fight through good elimination, no spicy or fatty foods, plenty of liquids and *natural* Diuretics.

Digestion

You may be suffering from malnutrition, even if you are carefully supplying your body with all the essential nutrients. The absorption of these different elements is in direct proportion to the efficiency of the digestive system! If this is faulty, absorption is minimal: food is passed through the body only partially digested. Rather than a digestive breakdown through enzymes and acids, it undergoes a process of bacterial decomposition. Putrefactive bacteria do break down protein into amino-acids, but they also destroy the amino acids and produce poisons and poisonous gases.

Some of these are expelled in the stool, but others are reabsorbed. When starches and sugars are not digested properly, they ferment and are broken down into alcohol, water and poisons. We take it for granted that fermentation (from sugars and starches) and putrefaction (from proteins) is a necessary occurrence. But we are also a sick people with many digestive-related diseases. Should we not then learn from the many animals and the few humans who have regular bowel-movements with odorless stools — who never suffer from gas and bad breath? Bertrand Russell credited his long, healthy and creative life to the fact that he regularly and without the aid of laxatives, moved his bowels twice a day. There is no point in supplying the body with foodstuffs, if these cannot be utilized through digestion — if they rot and decompose instead of yielding up their nutrients and calories. Bacterial activity is aided if digestion is impaired and if the gastric juices are not poured on the different elements at the proper time.

Factors which disturb or reduce digestive power are:

1. Emotional upset: anger, worry, anxiety, "butterflies".
2. Fatigue: rest after work, before eating, and rest after eating, before work.
3. Overeating — or eating too fast.
4. Poor food combinations (see Day 10, page 91).
5. Eating while ill, with fever and inflammations, or when in pain.
6. Eating when you are not hungry.
7. Vitamin-B deficiency (shown in a thickly-coated tongue or other tongue changes). This vitamin produces valuable bacteria in the intestine and the tongue symptoms usually point towards putrefaction in the intestine.
8. Hydrochloric acid deficiency — glutamic acid hydrochloride tablets and tablets of digestive enzymes could relieve your distress, says nutritionist Adelle Davis in LET'S EAT RIGHT TO KEEP FIT.'
9. Airswallowing — sip all cold drinks through a straw.
10. Insufficient protein supply, — since enzymes are made of protein and enzymes are only poured upon food if adequate protein is present. (Constipation may be caused by the poor muscle tone of the digestive tract brought about by the lack of protein). However, in modern society, usually *too much* protein is eaten.

KAREEN'S NUTRITIOUS WEIGHT LOSS DIET

MENU FOR DAY 11

Breakfast	½ chopped banana on ¼ cup crunchy Granola-type cereal, or Bircher Muesli* with small amount of skim milk.
Mid-morning	6 apricot halves (dried) **or** ½ cantaloupe
Lunch	1 tsp. yeast flakes **or** 1 tsp. soyflour in 1 cup orange juice 1 poached egg on one cup steamed, well-drained spinach
Mid-afternoon	1 medium apple **or** ½ cantaloupe
Dinner	2 cups tossed salad greens with ½ tbsp. oil & vinegar dressing ½ cup crab meat or shrimp 6 chilled asparagus spears sprinkled with lemon juice 1" square cheddar or gruyere cheese or muenster cheese.
Bedtime snack	10 almonds or 2 tsp. pinenuts or 2 tsp. pumpkin seeds.

* See recipe section

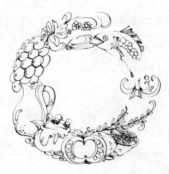

THIGHS

Today's breathing exercise is **The Humming Breath** which is excellent for insomnia and calming the nerves.

1. Perform a **Complete Breath** (see Day 3, page 28).
2. The second time make a soft humming sound while exhaling through the nose, with lips barely touching.
3. Repeat 3 - 10 times, sounding like a persistent bee.

The Side-Raise — firms and reduces fat in the thighs, hips and buttocks as well as benefitting the entire pelvic area.

Technique:

1. Lie on your right side, legs together, the right arm outstretched slightly in front of the head.
2. Raise the head and support it with your right palm covering half the ear. Place the left hand, palm down, just in front of the chest. (Figure 92)
3. Push down on the left hand and use the leverage to slowly raise the left leg as far as it will go. Keep the body in a straight line and both knees straight. (Figure 93)

(Figure 92)

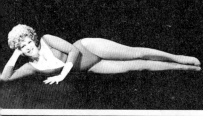

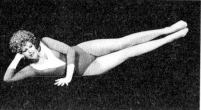

(Figure 94)

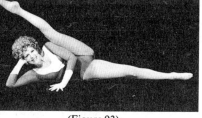

(Figure 93)

103

4. Hold the pose for 5 - 20 seconds, breathing normally.
5. EXHALE, lower the leg slowly and relax.
6. Now exhale and lift both legs together, the knees and ankles touching. (Figure 94)
7. Repeat on the other side.

Do's and Don'ts:

DO have the body in a completely straight line throughout. There is a tendency to stick the bottom out when the leg is raised high.
DO move as slowly in lowering the leg as you did in bringing it up.
DO NOT force beyond the point of comfort.

The Deep Lunge — strengthens and firms the thighs and calves while it develops balance and poise for the whole body.

Technique:

1. Stand, the feet about 2½ feet apart.
2. Turn the right foot to a 90° angle to the body, the left foot pointing straight forward. (Figure 95)
3. Bend your right knee and shift the body weight onto the right leg.
4. EXHALE, clasp your hands behind your back and bend the body forward, resting the chest on the right thigh. (Figure 96)
5. At the same time, slide the left leg back as far as possible, keeping the knee straight.
6. Having established your balance, now slowly slide the chest off the thigh on the inside and attempt to bring the head (forehead) to the floor. (Figure 97)
7. Hold for 10 - 30 seconds, breathing normally.
8. EXHALE, straighten up slowly and relax.
9. Repeat on the other side. Repeat on both sides twice more.

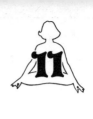

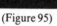
(Figure 95)

(Figure 96)

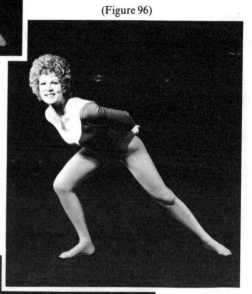
(Figure 97)

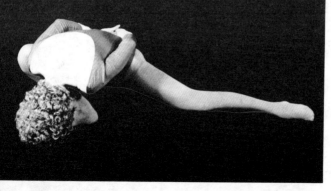

105

Do's and Don'ts:

DO keep the left foot pointed forward to give you a broader base of balance.

DO use the hands as support at the beginning.

DO use your body weight to help you bring the head closer to the floor, rather than jerking or forcing.

DO NOT bend your left knee.

The Forehead to Heel — works particularly on the outer thighs. Aiming the nose to the toes works on the inner thighs.

Technique:

1. Legs outstretched, pull one **heel** up beside the other knee.
2. Let the knee fall to the side. (Figure 98)
3. Join the two soles of the feet together.
4. Inhale, and clasp the fingers around the toes.
5. Exhale, and using the toes as leverage, pull yourself forward, aiming the forehead to the heels. Hold breathing normally for 5 - 30 seconds. (Figure 99)
6. Come up inhaling.
7. *Variation:* aim nose to the toes the next time (Figure 100)

Other poses that work on the thighs are:
Arm and Leg Stretch (Day 4, page 37)
Inclined Plane (Day 5, page 50)
Spread Leg Stretch Standing (Day 12, page 113)

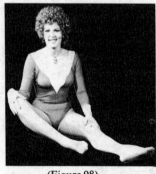
(Figure 98)

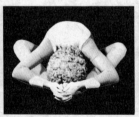
(Figure 99)

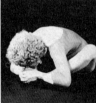
(Figure 100)

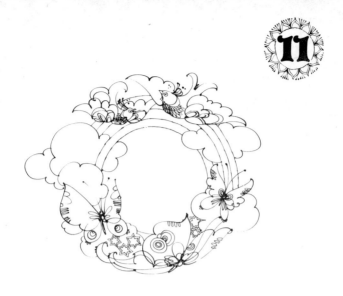

A SENSE MEDITATION

Please sit comfortably, with your spine straight, your head supported, and your feet up, in a quiet and peaceful part of the house. Let this be a meditation corner, your little retreat, where you come for the refreshing and relaxing qualities of meditation. Close your eyes; fold your hands; take one, two or three deep breaths, settle back and let go. Relax. Imagine that you are walking on the sand at the seaside. Drifting away from you into the horizon, until it blends with it, is the ever-changing ocean. The stretch of beach is endless and there is no one in sight. You have escaped. You welcome a feeling of solitude, of being alone. You amble along with your shoes in your hand, every step a sensation. You look at the blueness of the sky. It is interspersed now and then with fluffy little white clouds. You are at peace with nature. Feel the sand; feel it running through your toes; feel the warmth; be one with the sand every time you make a step; sink into it; unite with it. As you walk, feel the gentle breeze stroking against you, like a cat, soft, caressing, pleasantly cooling. Be a part of the wind, let it give of itself to you.

And now you tire. You sit down and pick up a conch shell lying in the sand, the inside white and smooth as alabaster. You take it in your hand, feel it, weigh it, look at it, sniff its salty odour and put it up to your ear. You hear the ocean — the rise and fall of the heaving waves, as they spend themselves on the wet sand, an eternal sound. As you listen, as the sound enters your ear and becomes part of your mind, you, too, want to be a part of this eternity, of the everlasting rise and fall of the waves. You put down the conch shell. You stand up, rid yourself of excess clothing and slowly enter the ocean. As you feel the warm waves rising around your body, as you submerge yourself in the velvety smoothness of the water, you become one with a rhythm of life that goes on eternally. The waves gently lift and hold you; you become weightless, you float, totally secure as in a womb. You are in nature's womb; you are part of the waves; you are part of the ocean; you *are* the waves; you *are* the ocean. You drift off. Seen from the beach, you become smaller and smaller, floating away into the horizon, to the line where heaven and earth meet, where the sun is setting in brilliant light, in purity and serenity. You drift towards the sun where the water joins with the horizon to become the universe. You welcome the feeling of diminishing size as you turn from an entity into a molecule, from a molecule to ether, becoming part of the blue and never-ending sky, part of the light, the truth and the knowledge of God's universe.

Day 12

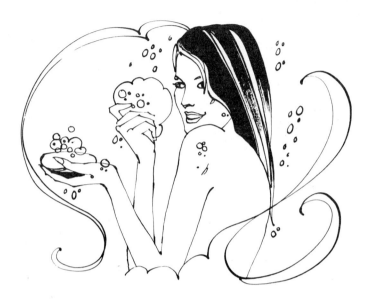

HEALTH PROBLEMS – BATH

What You Should Know!

— The use of water for beauty is ages old. But the use of the bath, as practised in the western world today, is also the greatest contributing factor for feminine infections.
— Today, informed doctors advise strongly against the use of a bath for women unless they have a cleansing shower in a separate stall first, as the orientals do.
— In the shower, the dirt that has been so assiduously scrubbed off, does not converge in a ring around the neck, or enter body openings or small wounds.
— Just soaking in the bath has great powers to relax or pep us up. It improves the circulation by stimulating the very small capilleries, veins and arteries to carry new food and beauty to the skin.
— When cleansing the body, scrubbing with a rough, fibrous cloth and with a pumice stone helps to shed scaly, dead cells.

What You Can Do!

1. To forestall urinary and bladder infection, one should never bathe or go swimming immediately after eliminating water.
2. The dye in toilet paper can be very irritating to delicate mucous membranes. Use white tissue.
3. If the skin is known to be sensitive, the use of water alone is sufficient to cleanse; soap is irritating. There is such a thing as being overly-clean. Beneficial bacteria, which ward off infection in the mucous membranes, are washed away.
4. Little girls should learn to take showers as early as they can.
5. Vitamin E has reportedly corrected vaginal inflammation, diaper rash and even teenage acne.
6. Vitamin D, the nerve relaxer, energy-maker, tooth and bone former and catalyst of the calcium family, is produced by ultraviolet light in sunshine from the oils *on* the skin (many people mistakenly think it is Vitamin C). However, the oil must be there, then be exposed to the short rays of the sun which reach us only in summer, and later be absorbed back into the body. So, it becomes very important that a bath is not taken several hours before or after sun-exposure.
7. Apart from polluting the atmosphere with gases escaping from aerosol cans, deodorant sprays are bad for our breathing passages. Vaginal deodorants are totally unnecessary. An excellent simple deodorant is a tablespoon of soda bicarbonate (baking soda) patted under each arm.
8. Give yourself a quick splashdown of apple cider vinegar from a cup. Oil yourself with the sweet-smelling sesame oil.

Combining Foods to make Proteins

To provide the body with complete proteins you could eat various types of meat or fish. However, vegetarians say that when eating meat you are consuming three times as much food as is necessary, since it takes at least that much vegetable matter to produce one animal. Vegetables can provide protein much more economically.

By careful selection you can combine certain vegetables to create complete proteins. So long as the combinations contain the 8 essential amino acids, the body can manufacture the other 14 amino acids needed by the body. A peanut butter sandwich comprises a complete protein because, although the peanut is a good source of protein it lacks some of the 8 basic amino acids which the whole wheat grain in the bread provides. Were one to eat the bread first, however, and the peanut butter an hour later, any benefits would be nullified. It is interesting to note here that sunflower seeds are a 'complete protein' source and that half a cup of these contributes more valuable protein (35 g.) than a five-ounce steak (30 g.) since muscle meats have a lesser quantity of each of the essential amino acids.

Some other foods that combine (in the same meal) to form complete protein are:

Grains with nuts
Beans with grains
* Brown rice with milk
Brown rice with beans
Brown rice with brewer's yeast
* Peanuts with milk
Peanuts with soy beans
* Sesame seeds with milk
Sesame seeds with beans
Sesame seeds with brown rice
* Potatoes with milk
* Beans with milk

* *Instead of 1 cup milk you may substitute:*
1/3 c. grated cheese, or
1/4 c. cottage cheese, or
1/3 c. ricotta, or
1/4 c. non-instant milk powder.

111

KAREEN'S NUTRITIOUS WEIGHT LOSS DIET

MENU FOR DAY 12

Breakfast	Fruit cup, 1 orange and ½ grapefruit
	2 tbsp. cottage cheese or quark
	1 slice dry pumpernickel toast
Mid-morning	1 tbsp. peanut butter
Lunch	1 cup fruit yogurt
	1 tbsp. hulled sunflower seeds
	or Pineapple Blender Drink:
	1 cup pineapple juice
	1 tbsp. non-instant skim milk powder
	1 tsp. yeast powder
	1 tsp. raw wheat germ
	1 egg
Mid-afternoon	3 cm. (1") square cheddar or muenster or gruyere cheese
Dinner	1 cup steamed broccoli
	1 cup steamed parsnips
	1 cup steamed carrots
	3 oz. lean roast beef
Bedtime snack	1 apple

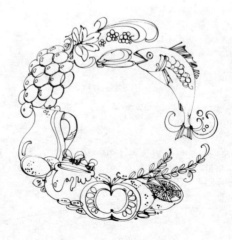

LEGS

Today's breathing exercise is **The Legs-up Breath** which is excellent for respiratory problems and for tired feet.

1. Lie on your back, buttocks against a wall, legs up. Cross the ankles, if you like.
2. Keep the arms on the floor but place them above the head, palms up, elbows straight.
3. Perform the **Complete Breath** three times, increasing the number to ten gradually.
4. *For tired feet* — lie as above and visualize immersing your feet into a red hot river when inhaling, then plunging them into a cool green lake when exhaling.

The Spread Leg Stretch Standing — stretches and develops the leg muscles, makes the legs shapely, and improves circulation to the upper body.

Technique:

1. Stand with the feet as wide apart as possible (1½ metres or 1-2/3 yards). (Figure 101)
2. INHALE, and place the hands at the waist, EXHALE, and bend slowly forward from the waist, keeping the back arched back.
3. When the body is parallel to the floor, bring the hands down in line with the feet, fingers pointing forward. (Figure 102)
4. INHALE and bring the head up.
5. EXHALE, bend the elbows, and aim the top of the head towards the floor in line with the hands. (Figure 103)
6. Hold the pose for 10 - 30 seconds, breathing deeply.
7. EXHALE, straighten up and relax. Repeat if necessary.

Do's and Don'ts:

DO keep the knees absolutely straight by tightening the knee caps.
DO have the feet, the hands and the top of the head all in a line.
DO NOT bend the back forward but keep a concave curve.
DO try to touch the head to the floor, eventually.

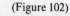
(Figure 102)

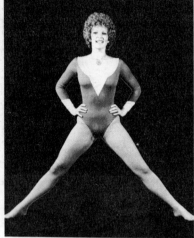
(Figure 101)

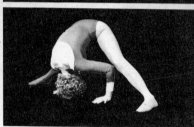
(Figure 103)

The Eagle — strengthens the ankles, legs and thighs and is useful to remove leg cramps.

Technique:

1. Stand, feet together, arms up at the sides for balance.
2. Bend the left knee and lift the right leg, bringing the right thigh over the left thigh as high up as possible, one against the other.
3. With the right calf pressed against the side of the left knee, bring the right foot around the back of the left leg and try to curl the right toes around the left ankle. (Figure 104)
4. Now bring the arms forward and bring the left arm over the right arm above the elbows.
5. Bend the right elbow and bring the right wrist over the left wrist, joining the hands. (Figure 105)
6. Balance in this position for 5 - 15 seconds, breathing normally.
7. OR, bend your body slowly forward from the waist, with the clasped hands in front of the face, until the elbows touch the knee. (Figure 106)
8. Disengage yourself, relax. Repeat on the other side.

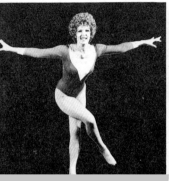
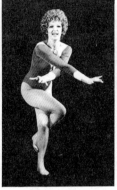
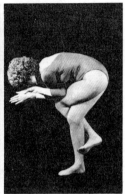

| (Figure 104) | (Figure 105) | (Figure 106) |

Do's and Don'ts:

DO practise simple balancing exercises first, if you have difficulty.
DO concentrate fiercely.
DO cross the legs up high, for an easier wrapping motion.
DO cross the arms in an opposite direction from the legs.
DO NOT attempt to bend forward until you are secure in the first part of the position

---

The Squat — is an excellent pose to do anytime because the toes are strengthened; the knee is exercised; varicose veins can be prevented.

Technique:

1. Stand with the feet slightly apart.
2. Raise the hands over your head and place the palms together.
3. Slowly rise up on your toes. (Figure 107)
4. Again, very slowly, bend your knees and start lowering your body. (Figure 108)
5. Continue down until you are resting on your heels.(Figure 109)
6. Do not hold. Very slowly push yourself all the way up until you are on the tips of your toes again.
7. Stay on your toes and repeat the overhead squat five times without pause.

115

Do's and Don'ts:

DO the overhead squats very slowly to derive the most benefit for
    your legs.
DO squat on your toes or heels whenever you can, i.e. while
    telephoning, peeling potatoes, etc.

Other effective poses for developing shapely and healthy legs
are:

Dog Stretch (Day 4, page 38)
Frog (Day 13, page 123)
Toe Twist (Day 13, page 124)

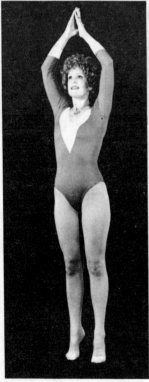
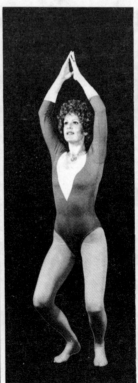
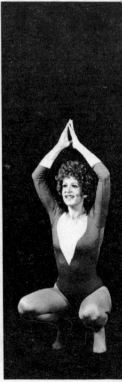

(Figure 107)   (Figure 108)   (Figure 109)

COMPUTER

You can learn to control your mind, just as surely as the mind now controls you. The mind is a source of energy which has barely been tapped. The reins for its control get stronger every time you *practise* meditation, and as you improve, you can make your mind work for you. A practical application of this is problem-solving.

Man's nervous system is extremely complex. Networks of nerve cells, some with fibers several feet long, run throughout the body, connecting every distant bit of tissue with the 10 billion nerve cells of the governing brain. Electrical impulses travel along these pathways at speeds ranging from 2 to 200 miles an hour, leaping across narrow gaps between cells, relaying intelligence to and from the brain. Just like a computer? Wrong. Instead, a computer is a very, very simplified version of the brain! But that brings up an interesting supposition. If a simple computer can give us answers to questions and problems, why can't we consciously use the much more sophisticated brain to do the same thing and more for us. All we have to do is to supply the data — the conscious data. Unconsciously, the brain has already collected and stored a considerable amount of information and impressions. It is the memory of what it has learned that the brain uses later on to help solve problems. My husband and I once had to spend considerable time commuting back and forth to work over a period of six months. To make the time pass more interestingly, we amused ourselves trying to work out the problem "What is intelligence?" After considerable argument, we came up with this definition: "Intelligence is the ability to adapt to new situations on the basis of past experience."

Today, consciously give your very own computer, your brain, *all* the available data you have on any given problem. Be careful to present both sides of the question. Do this at night in bed, just before you go to sleep. Lay it all on the line. Say, "Here's the problem, computer, here are all the facts. Now *you* work it out while I wash my hands of it and have a restful, worriless sleep." Then do just that. Relax, go to sleep. You'll be surprised how very often, some time during your day, the answer to your question, the decision or the solution "just comes to you". This is the power of a mind trained by concentration, contemplation, meditation.

Day 13

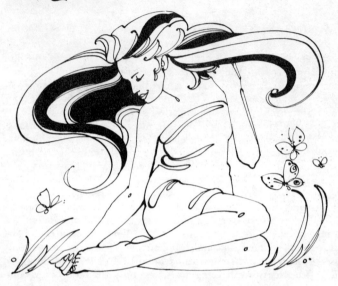

FOOT-CARE

What You Should Know!

— Every time a woman in high heels takes a step, she contacts the floor with a pressure of one ton per square inch, whereas a man of double her weight with *ordinary* shoes uses only 28 pounds of pressure per square inch. (And yet, for the most part, men design our shoes!)

— In each foot there are 26 delicate bones (more than half of our body's bones are situated in the hands and feet), 214 ligaments and thin bundles of muscles. Yet all together, with perfect padding and ridges, this foot, on a very small surface, balances the rest of our body most efficiently.

— The feet also contain myriads of tiny capillaries. The nerve endings on the bottom of the feet and toes correspond to various organs of the body. According to a new study called reflexology (a relative of acupuncture) some glands become sluggish due to wrong living and the contraction and relaxation of every cell that is constantly on-going in the body, is lessened.

— Reflexology divides the body into 10 zones, with all the nerves

118

ending in the feet and hands. When pressure is applied to an area of the foot which is the nerve reflex of a given part of the body, tenderness is felt in the foot. This soreness is due to crystalline deposits in the nerve ends and the poor circulation caused thereby. The congestion can be relieved and the affected organ can resume its normal function by *expert* application of pressure, say the reflexologists.

— Massage, as we have known for thousands of years, plays a very vital part in improving circulation and therefore beauty. By all means massage your feet often and vigorously, but leave reflexology itself, to the experts.

What You Can Do!

1. There are excellent foot-health shoes on the market and it is well worth your money to invest in a pair of them. They give good support, a revitalizing massage with every step. Otherwise, moccasins are good.
2. Use your fancy shoes for sitting prettily with ankles (not knees) crossed, at tea parties, and invest in healthy (no painful, strained, tired expression) shoes whenever you must walk.
3. Tilting the pelvis forward like a model while standing or walking, is healthy on both back and feet.
4. Insoles cushion the blow; changing into a second pair of shoes halfway through the day, gives a delightful "breather" to the feet.
5. Headaches? Make an outline of your bare foot on a piece of paper, then one of your shoes over top. Shoes too small?
6. Walking along the outside edge of the foot, from heel to little toe, is the least stressful to the foot.
7. Foot and leg cramps in pregnancy can be corrected by Vitamin B-6. Calcium in a glass of milk — with 2 or 3 extra calcium tablets if it's a severe case — before exercise, is a good idea for muscle-cramps. It soothes nerves as well.
8. Tired feet? A cold footbath in which you step up and down on your toes is an effective ballerina trick.
9. Varicose veins? Make a habit of "whipping" up on your toes in an exaggerated manner whenever you go up *any* stairs. It encourages calf-muscle action to help push the blood straight up. Otherwise: legs up, up, up whenever possible.

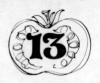

Miracle Foods to add to the Family Diet

To round out your daily diet do become familiar with these easily obtained "extra" foods which, in concentrated, natural form, make your search for good family nutrition a breeze.

Almonds — good source of magnesium, iron and protein. Contains Laetril, which is now used for cancer therapy. Good to rid the system of intestinal parasites when eaten with figs.

Apple Cider Vinegar — is said to be effective for weight-control, bleeding (has a beneficial blood-clotting effect in preventing profuse bleeding after operations, such as tonsillectomies), to offset food poisoning and diarrhea, to ease the pain of arthritis, sore throat and laryngitis, to act as a soporific with insomnia, to help with asthma, and vertigo. One teaspoon per day in a glass of water, or serve as salad dressing.

Brewer's Yeast — one to two tablespoons in fruit juices or warm water with meals. If a B-vitamin deficiency is suspected, this dosage can gradually be stepped up to 3 - 4 tbsp. a day. It is quite palatable and soluble in flake form, undetectable in meat loaf, stews, cereals, soups. Your very deficiency will express itself by gas at first, until corrected; so persist.

Dessicated Liver — is fresh liver dried at low temperatures to preserve the precious vitamins, minerals and proteins; is available in tablet or powder form; contains all the B-vitamins in proper balance which makes assimilation easy and complete; is a perfect substitute or complement for Brewer's Yeast — take them together or by itself for pure blood and good health.

Garlic — is a natural antibiotic and general blood purifier. By providing the body with phosphorus and potassium it can correct blood pressure problems, asthma, rheumatism and skin eruptions. It is disliked by intestinal parasites in pearl-form or if used in enema-water for four consecutive days.

Kelp — is a good source of protein, iodine, calcium and magnesium. Use it as a substitute for salt by getting the powdered form. It is available in tablet form also.

Lecithin — especially if there is a record of heart disease or high cholesterol. The phosphorus of protein foods, and fats, help

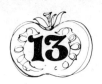

to form it. Keeps skin and nerves young and healthy. Found in glandular meat such as heart, kidney, brain, in egg yolk, soy beans and lecithin granules.

Molasses *(unsulphured)* — one or two teaspoons in milk, muffins, cookies, other baking, or in casseroles or as a sleep cocktail, for iron, calcium, B-vitamins, or simply as a laxative. Also available in powdered form in health food stores.

Wheat germ *and/or* **wheat germ oil** — the former enriches all baked goods and is considered the best cereal because of B-vitamins, protein, iron and Vitamin E content. Should be kept in refrigerator and can be sprinkled on cereals, added to blender drinks, or put into baking and casseroles.

KAREEN'S NUTRITIOUS WEIGHT LOSS DIET

MENU FOR DAY 13

Breakfast	Fruit cup: 1 orange, ½ grapefruit ½ cup canned tuna 1 slice pumpernickel toast **or** 1 muffin ½ pat butter
Mid-morning	1 banana **or** ½ cantaloupe

Lunch	Orange blender drink:
	   1 cup orange juice
	   2 tsp. vanilla soy protein powder
	   or 2 tbsp. non-instant skim milk powder
	   1 tsp. powdered yeast
	   1 egg

Mid-afternoon	1 tbsp. peanut butter or ½ cup peanuts
Dinner	2 poached eggs 1 slice light rye toast 1 pat butter

Bedtime snack	1 chicken breast
	   or 1 slice roast beef
	   or 1 hard-cooked egg.

FEET AND ANKLES

Today's breathing exercise is **The Cleansing Breath**, to tone the nervous system and purify the bloodstream.

1. Sit in a comfortable cross-legged position or a chair, back straight.
2. Inhale deeply, pushing the abdomen out, and taking in as much air as possible in the space of 1 second.
3. Whack your abdomen in forcefully to expel the air through the nostrils. The sensation should be one of having been punched in the stomach.
4. Inhale again by pushing the abdomen out and letting the air rush back into the vacuum created by the exhalation.
5. The whole process, inhalation and exhalation, should take not much more than 1½ seconds. Both should be forceful and will be quite audible.
6. Repeat ten times, follow with a complete breath and repeat ten times more.

The Ankle Bends — relieve swollen ankles and feet and strengthen weak ankles.

Technique:

1. Stand straight, feet 6 cm. apart. (2 inches)
2. Roll to the right onto the sides of your feet. (You will be resting on the outside of the right foot and on the inside of the left foot. (Figure 110)
3. Bend your knees forward and to the right, but keep your hips and pelvis to the front.
4. Hold the position for 5 seconds or until you begin to be uncomfortable.
5. Repeat on the other side.
6. Sit down with your knees drawn up.
7. Let the right leg stretch straight out in front while the other rests in the crock of the left arm. (Figure 111)
8. With both hands manipulate the left foot; work the ankle in a clockwise direction, then reverse it. Repeat rotations three times. (Figure 112)
9. "Play" with the toes, massage the heel and the whole sole.
10. Change feet and repeat 8 and 9.

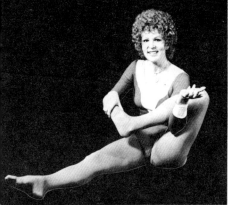

(Figure 111)

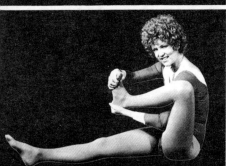
(Figure 112)

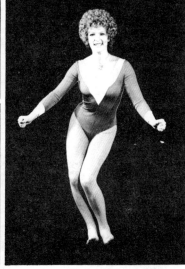
(Figure 110)

Do's and Don'ts:

DOing the exercises regularly will keep a youthful spring in your step, as stiff ankles are one of the first signs of old age.

DON'T swivel your pelvis to the side — you would waste your effort.

The Frog — helps flat feet, softens calcaneal spurs, relieves pain in the heels, and removes fatigue from the legs and feet.

Technique:

1. Lie on the floor, face down. Bring the hands, palms down, under the shoulders.
2. Bend the RIGHT knee and bring the heel close to the buttocks. (Figure 113)
3. Place the space between index finger and thumb of the right hand on *top* of the right foot, the thumb pointing towards the body. The elbow *must* point straight up to the ceiling.
4. EXHALE, lift your head and shoulders off the floor, looking up, and press down on the foot, pushing it towards the floor.

123

5. Hold the pose from 10 - 30 seconds, breathing normally. (Figure 114)
6. EXHALE, lower the body and relax.
7. Repeat with the other foot. Try it with both feet, when ready. (Figure 115)

Do's and Don'ts:

DO be sure to place the hands properly on the feet. The motion is one of pushing down rather than pulling down.

DO prepare for the **Frog** with such exercises as the **Sitting and Reclining warrior**, the **Japanese Sitting Position** and the **Lotus**.

DO follow the breathing instructions accurately.

DO NOT force the feet down beyond comfort.

(Figure 113)

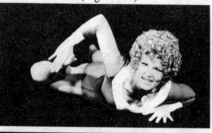

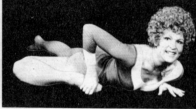

(Figure 114)

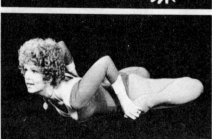

(Figure 115)

Other poses that are excellent for developing feet and leg muscles and "oiling" the knees and ankles are:

Dog Stretch (Day 4, page 38)
Ear to Knee (Day 7, page 66)
Squat (Day 12, page 115)

The Toe Twist — strengthens feet and ankles, improves balance and makes legs shapely.

Technique:

1. Stand erect with your feet together, toes slightly pointed outward.

124

2. Come slowly up on your toes, at the same time bringing both hands together in front of you, arms straight, thumbs interlocking, palms down. (Figure 116)
3. Keep your eyes riveted on the backs of your hands for better balance.
4. Slowly bring the arms as far as you can to the side, twisting from the waist and keeping the toes firmly dug in. (Figure 117)
5. Hold 10 - 20 seconds. Slowly return to the front.
6. Repeat on the other side. Repeat twice more to both sides. (Figure 118)

Do's and Don'ts:

DO NOT become distracted if you lose your balance. Simply try again.
DO NOT in any way allow your toes to swivel as you twist.
DO keep your body straight, chest out.

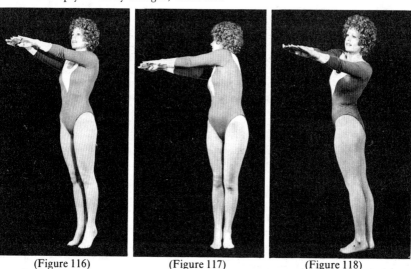

(Figure 116)   (Figure 117)   (Figure 118)

Goal Attainment

The Yogi speaks always of a trinity of beings, which make up the whole man: the body, the mind and the soul (or spirit).

125

Through Hatha Yoga we exercise the body, through meditation we train the mind and by working on both of these we elevate the level of our spirit. To reach a higher level of awareness we must first be able to *control* the mind. It must be taught to put away fear and anxiety and distrust, to have faith in the universal law of love and to send out positive vibrations through the chanting of the OM or through the mental repetition of an ennobling thought.

Man is both a transmitter and a receiver in the cosmos. His every deed, his every thought "sends" and is "received". This is why positive thinking is so important. The long life of a 99-year-old woman in Canada who practises Yoga may be due to her outlook on life: "Every morning I will say something happy will come my way." She is sending out positive thoughts and the people who are receptive to them, receive them. This way something happy DOES come her way. She has FAITH. Conversely, I know a man who always expects to be disappointed by life, by other people, by luck and he IS! The bible says, "Ask, and ye shall receive."

Is goal-attainment as opposed to wishfulfillment or daydreaming, really possible? The Yogi believes that you can set yourself a goal and expect it to be fulfilled through an act of faith. It is necessary, here, to set out the "ten commandments" of Yoga. They are called Yamas and Niyamas. They consist of five abstinences: non-violence, truthfulness, non-stealing, chastity and non-receiving; and five observances: purity (both inner and outer), contentment, austerity, study and worship of God. This immediately precludes your visualizing anything negative or harmful to others. Indeed, to bless a naughty child, to wish a difficult neighbour well, to love an infected finger, is to start a wonderful healing process in the object and in your own mind. It will show in added beauty and serenity to your face and personality. How is visualizing a goal different from prayer? In one you ask for enlightenment and knowledge, in the other, you *live* that which in your heart, you visualize fulfilled. That is, you cannot ask for health and yet think and speak illness; you cannot visualize wealth and live inactively and poorly organized; you cannot expect to keep receiving when you do not give — of yourself or through a tithe or by giving thanks for what you have received.

The steps for goal attainment are exactly proscribed: 1. Know exactly what you want and be sure that you *really* want it. 2. Visualize, in all its details, that it already exists, has already happened. 3. Give thanks.

126

Day 14

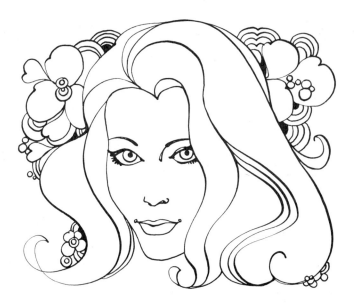

EYES

What You Should Know!

— The eyes are probably the most often used organ of your body.
— Your eyes are the only true spot of colour in your entire body, a most important fact in making you the individual you are.
— The six muscles in each eye make for high mobility and help to make it the most eloquent part of your face.
— The eyes are like perfect little machines, which work chemically, and which therefore need the whole gamut of vitamins and minerals and amino acids (proteins) to purr along satisfactorily.
— When a nutritional deficiency exists, the eyes are one of the first to suffer and dull, bloodshot, itchy, short or long sighted eyes peer out on the world.
— If your eyes hurt, when you meet the bright lights of an oncoming car at night for example, you may be suffering from an A-Vitamin deficiency.

What You Can Do!

1. For a sensitivity to lights and for a feeling that mere dimness or dusk is real darkness, vitamins A and B-2 will help to improve seeing in the dark and give you shiny, healthy eyes.

2. Dried and fresh apricots are an excellent source of vitamin A and iron. Children love them in lunch-boxes and they are very tasty eaten with almonds.

3. Vitamin C helps to strengthen capilleries. Vitamin B-2 is also very helpful with bloodshot, itching, burning eyes.

4. The greatest beautifier of all: lots of sleep.

5. Puffy eyes, face and hands in the morning and puffy ankles by the end of the day are one of the symptoms of protein deficiency. What to do? Soothing applications of camomile tea to the whole eye area.

6. There are many indications that fluorescent lights should be avoided.

7. Eyelash lengtheners? Dip your little mascara brush into a protein rich polypeptide liquid solution. Or, try applying coconut oil or castor oil to the eyelashes and brows.

8. Refreshers? Cold-water washcloth applications, a rinsing of the eyes with a solution of boric acid in boiled water, or giving a good kneading, gently-pinching massage to the back of the neck. Try them: the old fashioned remedies will work best.

9. To relax uptight muscles? First, warm water application, then eye exercise, always followed by palming.

10. Tired eyes – black circles? Try used rose hip tea bags, or cucumber slices, or raw grated potatoes in a cheesecloth on the eyes. Other factors for the circles could be lack of fresh air, exercise, intestinal parasites or constipation.

11. The best position? On a slantboard while doing eye exercises or applications. If a 99 year-old clear-eyed, clear-headed lady in Canada can do a perfect shoulderstand and plough on a slantboard, so can you!

12. Crepey look under the eyes and on neck? Try odorless castor oil; always be gentle and always stroke *down* on the neck.

13. Be gentle when applying only light creams and oils to the delicate eye area. Sticky creams drag and stretch. Use your third finger, look up, work outward over the eyelids, then inward toward the nose. Use little circular motions at the corner.

14. Be careful not to put too much oil under the eyes — it can smudge up, irritate and puff up the eyes overnight.

Menstruation

There is a reason why so many women become "witches" before their periods. It has to do with the blood calcium level. This drops steadily for about ten days, causing pre-menstrual tension, headaches, "nerves", insomnia, and water retention. Some women gain up to 10 pounds during this time. Others find their resistance to allergies and infection lessened. Adelle Davis advises calcium tablets (containing magnesium) and vitamin D (to ensure better absorption of the calcium) for at least a week before menstruation, and for a year before puberty — another time when blood calcium drops considerably. For uterine cramps on the first day, take one or two tablets of calcium every hour. Often, menstrual difficulties — and water retention — disappear if 1 - 2 tbsp. of vegetable oil (linoleic acid) are taken daily. The lack of vitamin B-12 (only found in meat, cheese, eggs and milk) may also cause problems, especially in vegetarians who do not carefully combine their proteins.

Water Retention

Water retention should be corrected by first determining the cause. Diuretics do not solve the problem permanently and do irreparable damage in the meantime. Water, combined with sodium, passes into the cells in the first place because a lack of potassium has permitted this. Diuretics, coffee and alcohol only aggravate the deficiency problem through increased urine production, since potassium, magnesium and other valuable water-soluble nutrients are lost in the urine. Much better to correct the problem through a good diet of adequate protein, potassium (bananas, apple cider vinegar, cantaloupes, peanuts and potassium chloride tablets), vitamin C and the essential fatty acids (1 - 2 tbsp. of vegetable oils a day). These will help you to lose many watery pounds *safely*.

Anemia

If you are energyless, feel weak, dizzy and short of breath; if you have a pounding heartbeat, palpitations and feelings of being

129

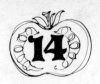

dead tired; if you look pale and listless, have brittle nails with longitudinal ridging, can't think clearly and forget easily — you may well be suffering from anemia. Check with your doctor. He may tell you to take extra iron. Excellent food sources of iron are: liver (especially pork liver), heart, kidney, lean meats, shell fish, egg yolk, dried beans, dried fruit (especially apricots), whole grain products, blackstrap molasses, brewer's yeast and wheat germ.

Only about 50% of iron is absorbed even by a healthy person. Generally, the softer the texture of the food, the better the absorption. Hydrochloric acid must dissolve iron before it can be absorbed, but most anemic persons lack this acid. Agents which help to ensure absorption are: B-vitamins (help to form hydrochloric acid), vitamin C, and acidic foods such as yogurt, buttermilk, sour fruit and citric juices. Refined carbohydrates prevent absorption. Most iron salts destroy vitamin E, so that you should take your Vitamin E in the morning as an anti-stress agent, and your iron no less than 10 hours later. As always, good food sources rich in the missing element are better than supplementation.

Menopause

Why is it that some women sail smoothly through menopause, while others come close to a nervous breakdown or to causing one in those who have to live with them? To the healthy person, who is not "undernourished" due to deficiencies and whose glands are not run-down, menopause will mean nothing more or less than the end of her child-bearing years. The temporary readjustment and slowdown going on in the endocrine glands (particularly the gonads — ovaries, thyroid and pituitary) will quickly be adjusted to. These glands secrete their hormones directly into the bloodstream in adequate amounts. If the body has been well-nourished, says Lelord Kordel in *Health Through Nutrition,* vitamins A and C and certain proteins stimulate the ovaries. Vitamin E (staggering the amount gradually up to 400 or 500 i.u.'s daily) often helps to make hot flashes disappear and it is the vitamin which gives us our "curves". For nervous symptoms during the menopause, calcium (with magnesium and with Vitamin D to ensure absorption) is excellent because the lack of ovarian hormones causes severe calcium deficiency.

KAREEN'S NUTRITIOUS WEIGHT LOSS DIET

MENU FOR DAY 14

Breakfast	Pineapple blender drink:
	1 cup pineapple juice
	1 tbsp. non-instant skim milk powder
	1 tsp. yeast powder
	1 tsp. wheat germ (raw)
	1 egg
	or *breakfast described for Day 7*
Mid-morning	1 tbsp. honey
Lunch	¾ cup raw grated cabbage
	or ½ cup raw grated beets
	1 medium grated raw carrot
	1 chopped green onion
	½ cup alfalfa sprouts
	with 1 tbsp. oil and vinegar dressing
	1 buttered rye crisp
Mid-afternoon	1 banana
Dinner	1 cup French onion soup
	3 oz. ground round
	1 cup French string beans
	½ cup steamed carrots
	½ cup steamed spinach
Bedtime snack	8 almonds
	1 tbsp. sunflower seeds

RELAXATION

Today's poses should totally absorb your thoughts when you do them. The time spent on RELAXATION should not be shared with any other activity no matter how short a time you spend at RELAXING.

Today's breathing exercise is **The Warming Breath** to allow you to concentrate the benefits of prana (life-force) on a specific part of your body.

1. Sit with the legs crossed.
2. Inhale and then concentrate on a small area of the body; start with a palm or the index finger, for example.
3. Inhale and concentrate until there is a sensation of warmth on your chosen part of your body.
4. Exhale for the same length of time as the inhalation.

Do's and Don'ts:

DO try again and again until you achieve warmth in the chosen area before moving to a large "target".

DO use this method to warm your feet in winter.

DO NOT be discouraged if you do not succeed at once; it takes intense concentration to achieve warmth from breathing.

The Rock 'n Rolls — is an excellent warmup and energizer as it massages and reduces the tension in the spine and neck area.

Technique:

1. Sit on the floor, knees bent.
2. Clasp your hands under the knees.
3. Bring your head as close to the knees as possible and keep it there throughout. (Figure 119)
4. Rock gently back onto the spine, keeping the back rounded and the legs together. (Figure 120)
5. Establish an easy rhythm in rocking back and forth.
6. Repeat 12 times or up to a minute.
7. Remember to breathe in as you roll back, out as you come forward.
8. *Variation:* Cross your ankles and repeat steps 1 to 7. (Figure 121)

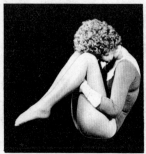
(Figure 119)

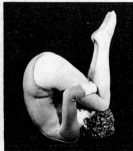
(Figure 120)

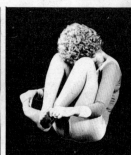
(Figure 121)

Do's and Don'ts:

DO start the whole exercise on your back if you are a bit timid about rocking back from a sitting position.

DO the **Rock 'n Rolls** any time you want to get the kinks out of your body.

DO keep your head close to your knees, to have a rounded spine to rock on.

DO use the momentum of the first backward rock to return forward again.

The Curling Leaf — eases tension because you assume the therapeutic position of pre-birth; it acts as a relaxer and an energizer at the same time.

Technique:

1. Kneel with legs together.
2. Rest your buttocks on the heels and the top of your hands on the floor, pointing back. (Figure 122)
3. Lower your head slowly to the floor, the hands sliding gently back, palms up, to lie beside the body. (Figure 123)
4. Rest your head on the forehead or turned to the side, on the floor and relax completely with the chest against the knees.
5. Hold for any length of time, the longer the better.

Do's and Don'ts:

DO the **Curling Leaf** any time you need a rest or a pick-up.

DO NOT stick your bottom up in the air but put your whole weight on your legs and heels.

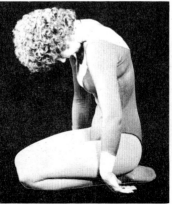

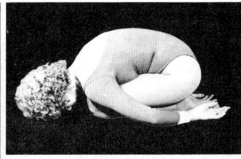

(Figure 123)

(Figure 122)

The Sponge — teaches one to relax the whole body and free it from anxiety, nervous tension, is an energy recharger.

Technique:

1. Lie on the floor, legs slightly apart, arms limply by your side. (Figure 124)
2. Point your toes away from you and hold for 5 seconds. Relax.
3. Pull the toes up towards the body, bending at the ankle.
4. Pull your heels up two inches off the floor and then straighten the legs, pushing the back of the knees firmly against the floor. Hold. Relax.
5. Point the toes toward each other and pull the heels under and up, keeping the legs straight. Hold. Relax.
6. Pinch your buttocks together. Hold. Relax.
7. Pull your abdomen in and up as far as possible. Hold. Relax.
8. Arch the spine back, pushing the chest out. Hold. Relax.
9. With arms straight by your side, palms down, bend the fingers up and back toward the arm, bending at the wrist. Hold. Relax.
10. Bend the elbows and repeat step 9, bending the hands back toward the shoulders. Hold. Relax. (Figure 125)
11. Make a tight fist of your hands, bring the arms out to the sides and move the arms up perpendicular to the floor. Move very slowly, resisting the movement all the while to make the pectoral muscles of the bust stand out.
12. Pull the shoulder blades of the back together. Hold. Relax.
13. Pull the shoulders up beside the ears. Hold. Relax.
14. Pull down the corners of the mouth. Hold. Relax.
15. Bring the tongue to the back of the roof of the mouth. Hold. Relax.
16. Purse your lips, wrinkle the nose and squeeze the eyes tightly shut. Hold. Relax.
17. Smile with the lips closed and stretch the face. Hold. Relax.
18. Yawn very slowly, resisting the movement.
19. Press the back of the head against the floor. Hold. Relax. (Figure 126)
20. Frown, moving the scalp forward. Hold. Relax.
21. Go through the eye exercises.
22. Pull your head under and against the shoulder without moving anything else.
23. Relax, melting into the floor, for up to 10 minutes. (Figure 124)

Do's and Don'ts:

DO hold each holding position for at least 5 seconds.

DO relax after each holding position, by flopping back into place after the flexing position.

DO NOT worry or think of unpleasant things as you relax at the end of the **Sponge**. Rather keep your thoughts to a minimum, on pleasant things, and dispassionately watch them wander past without trying to become involved.

Other poses that are excellent for relaxing certain parts of the body are:

The Lion (Day 1, page 11)
The Chest Expander (Day 6, page 56)
The Shoulderstand (Day 2, page 19)

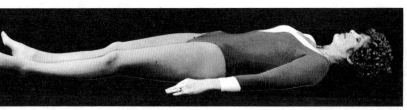

(Figure 124)

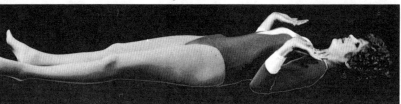

(Figure 125)

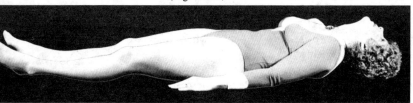

(Figure 126)

135

14 Thoughts to Contemplate — One for each Day

1. I will try to be happy under all circumstances. I will make up my mind to be happy within myself right now where I am today.

   .....Paramahansa Yogananda

2. Chance never helps those who do not help themselves.

   .....Sophocles

3. There is no cosmetic for beauty like happiness.

   .....Lady Blessington

4. Kindness is the golden chain by which society is bound together.

   .....Goethe

5. The physician heals, nature makes well. All art, all education can be merely a supplement to nature.

   .....Aristotle

6. I have buried dead disappointments in the cemeteries of yesterday. Today I will plow the garden of life with my new creative efforts.

   .....Paramahansa Yogananda

7. A feeble body weakens the mind.

   .....J.J. Rousseau

8. They can conquer who believe they can.

   .....Virgil

9. Humility is the solid foundation of all virtues.

   .....Confucius

10. Please do understand that every relation will deceive you in the long run except the relation of truth.

    .....Shyam

11. Knowledge comes but wisdom lingers.

    .....Tennyson

12. People seldom improve when they have no other model but themselves to copy after.

    .....Goldsmith

13. It is easier to suppress the first desire than to satisfy all that follow it.

    .....Franklin

14. Self-conquest is the greatest of victories.

    .....Plato

RECIPES IN THE DIET

Recipes Tested by Kareen

Bircher Apple Muesli

Simply soak overnight one level tablespoon of whole cereal in two tablespoons of water. Next morning, add the juice of half a lemon and one tablespoon of condensed milk, and mix. Quickly shred one large unpeeled apple into the mixture, and stir in a tablespoon each of honey and wheat germ. Serve at once. To increase the protein content you may also add a tablespoon of chopped walnuts almonds or sunflower seeds.

Easy Granola

9 cups raw oats	*¾ cup date sugar or honey*
2 cups soy flour	*½ cup oil mixed with*
1 cup whole wheat flour	*1 cup boiling water*
or wheat germ	*2 tsp. salt*
½ cup coconut, shredded	*1 tsp. vanilla*

Blend together liquid ingredients. Stir into dry ingredients. Crumble and bake on cookie sheets. Start at 350° for 15 minutes, then lower to 200° and bake until dry and golden brown. Keeps well. Store in covered jars.

Wheat Germ Muffins

1 cup unbleached flour or pastry wheat flour
1 cup whole wheat flour
3 tsps. no alum baking powder
½ tsp. salt
2 tbsp. honey
1 cup milk
1/3 cup vegetable oil
1 egg
½ cup wheat germ

Mix dry ingredients (except wheat germ) together. Mix moist ingredients together and stir into dry ingredients. Add wheat germ last. Bake at 350° for 20 mins. in greased muffin tins. Makes 12 muffins.

Yogurt I

1 cup whole milk
1 cup non-instant milk powder
3 tbsp. yogurt (commercial or your own culture)
3 cups warm water

Stir well and pour into pint jars, a big bowl, or special yogurt makers. Follow 3 simple rules and you will have yogurt in 3 to 8 hours ready for cooling and eating.
1.   Make certain all containers are very clean.
2.   Maintain the heat at 110° F.
3.   Do not disturb.
Alternate ways to maintain constant heat: a yogurt maker, electric food warmer, the oven at lowest heat, a heating pad, a down blanket or pillow, radiator, heating duct, pilot light of the gas stove, top of a radio or television set, or a thermos bottle.

Yogurt II

2 cups tepid water
1½ cups non-instant powdered skim milk
Yogurt culture
      or 3 tbsp. commercial or previously made yogurt

Pour mixture into a pitcher containing:

1 quart tepid water + 1 large can evaporated milk.

Stir well and pour into drinking glasses or pint jars. Set glasses or jars in dry yogurt maker. If yogurt maker is not used, put into large pan of warm water, bring water level to rim of glasses or jars, cover pan, and set over pilot light or in warming oven where a temperature of 100° to 120° F. can be maintained. For smaller amounts, heat the milk slightly, then pour mixture into a thermos bottle.
Check consistency at end of 3 hours. Chill immediately after the milk thickens. Yogurt will keep in the refrigerator for 5 days or longer.

Variations:

Serve with brown sugar and cinnamon, honey and finely shredded orange or lemon rind, or sweetened berries, peaches, other fresh fruit or canned applesauce or pineapple.

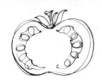

Pineapple Blender Drink

1 cup pineapple juice
1 tbsp. non-instant skim milk powder (or soy flour)
1 tsp. yeast powder
1 tsp. wheat germ (raw)
1 egg

Orange Blender Drink

1 cup orange juice
2 tsp. vanilla soy protein powder
*   OR 2 tbsp. non-instant skim milk powder*
1 tsp. powdered yeast
1 egg

Beet Borscht (Makes approximately 6 cups)

Chop very finely:
¾ cup carrots
1 cup onion
2 cups beets

Cover with small amount of water and simmer with lid on for 20 minutes. Then add:

1 tbsp. butter
2 cups beef or other stock
1 cup finely shredded cabbage (or sauerkraut)
1 tbsp. apple cider vinegar
1 sprig chopped parsley or dill

Season with garlic salt, bay leaf and fine herbs to suit taste. Simmer, covered, for additional 20 minutes.

Health Bread (Pegge Gabbott)

2 cups whole wheat flour
3 cups bran
2 tbsp. wheat germ
2 tbsp. rice polishings
2 tbsp. grated cheese
2 - 3 tbsp. sunflower seeds
½ tsp. celery seed (opt.)
½ tsp. caraway seed (opt.)
½ tsp. cumin seed (opt.)
½ tsp. flaxseed (opt.)
1 tsp. vegetable salt (or sea salt)
1 tsp. baking powder
1 tsp. baking soda *(or 2 tsp. baking powder*
2 tbsp. nutritional yeast

Mix:
1½ cups buttermilk
1 tbsp. Safflower oil (cold pressed)

Add to solids.
Mix, shape like round loaf, sprinkle with flour.
Bake 60 minutes at 350° F. on a cookie sheet.

Variation:

2 cups whole wheat flour and 1 cup graham flour or 3 cups graham flour.

Fruit Loaf:

Substitute honey and/or grated lemon or orange rind, and any kind of dried fruit, dates, figs, raisins, soaked apricots, for the spices.

Soybean Muffins

1 cup Soybean flour
2 tsp. no alum baking powder
1/8 tsp. baking soda
½ cup. chopped walnuts

½ tsp. vanilla
½ cup buttermilk
2 eggs, separated

Mix and sift dry ingredients; add nuts, beat egg yolks with vanilla, buttermilk and soda. Fold stiffly beaten egg whites. Bake in slow oven. Makes 12 muffins.

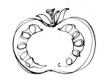

Carrot Cake

1½ cups Safflower salad oil — cold pressed
2 cups raw sugar
4 eggs

Mix salad oil and sugar. Then add eggs one at a time and mix after each.

2 cups whole wheat pastry flour (fine)
2 tsp. baking soda (sifted, then measured)
*   OR double baking powder instead of soda*
2 tsp. baking powder
2 tsp. cinnamon
1 tsp. salt
3 cups shredded carrot
1 cup chopped nuts (or flaked coconut)
1 can pineapple bits (optional, with one extra cup flour)

Sift the above dry ingredients together and slowly add the wet mixture, mixing well. Then add the carrots and nuts, mix, and pour into 3 separate oiled pans. Bake at 300° for 50 minutes or until done.

Frosting can be of your own choice; however a cream cheese frosting, made from the softened cheese and honey to taste, is delicious.

Bran Muffins

3 cups whole wheat flour
2 cups Bran
1 cup dry milk
3 tsp. baking powder
1 tsp. baking soda
1½ tsp. salt

Mix together, then add:

2 cups water
4 eggs
½ cup oil
½ cup molasses
¾ cup honey
1 cup dates OR raisins

Add *sunflower seeds*.

Batter is quite wet.
Bake at 350° for 15 - 20 minutes.
Do not overcook!

VITAMINS

BENEFITS	DEFICIENCY SYMPTOMS	FOOD SOURCES
A —VISION, SKIN, MUCOUS MEMBRANES, RESISTANCE TO INFECTION, GROWTH AND REPRODUCTION. Soluble in fats and oils, insoluble in water, not affected by heat, but loses activity if exposed to air at any time. Not affected by alkalies.	A —Night blindness and poor vision or sensitivity to light, dry, scaly skin, gallbladder and kidney stones, poor teeth, retarded growth, thinness, coarse or falling-out hair, pneumonia, inflammation of the reproductive organs, diarrhea, apathy and frequent infections and colds.	A —Green-pigment plants, the greener the better. —Yellow vegetables, peaches, persimmons, yams. —Fish liver oil, liver, egg yolks, milk, butter, cream. —Twice as much is needed when the Vit. A. is derived from carotene.
B¹ (Thiamin)—ENERGY, APPETITE, RESISTANCE TO INFECTION, DIGESTION (HYDROCHLORIC ACID). Soluble in water, insoluble in fats and oils, partially destroyed by pasteurization, intake should be increased when carbohydrates are increased.	B¹ —Slow then rapid pulse, short windedness (athletes need more), poor digestion (gas, constipation), craving for sweets, poor appetite, mental depression, anemia, poor sleep.	B¹ —In the seed: wheat germ, rice polishings, cereal grains, nuts, beans, peas, soy beans, lentils, unrefined bread products, liver (raw), heart, kidneys, brewer's yeast, oysters, barley, asparagus, parsley, raw apple, radish, watercress, lemon, grapefruit, celery, cabbage, carrots, pomegranate, coconut, dandelion.
B² (Riboflavin)—YOUTHFUL SKIN, VITALITY, LONGEVITY. Soluble in water, not affected by air or heat, destroyed by alkalies and sunlight.	B²—Dim vision, bloodshot and inflamed eyes, oily skin, sore cracked mouth, swollen eyelids.	B² —Liver, yeast, (butter) milk, leafy vegetables (outer leaves are five times better), yogurt, glandular meats, dairy products, raw crabmeat, broccoli, mushrooms, oysters, whole wheat flour, soy flour and beans, apple, apricot, carrot, coconut, dandelions, grapefruit, prune, spinach, watercress.

Vitamin / Function	Deficiency Symptoms	Food Sources
C —"BEAUTY AND YOUTH" vitamin, STRONG TEETH and BONES, RESISTANCE TO INFECTION, QUICK HEALING OF WOUNDS AND BROKEN BONES, SOOTHING AND BENEFICIAL DURING ANY ILLNESS, ANTITOXIC, PREVENTS FATIGUE. Soluble in water, insoluble in oils, not affected by heat except if exposed to oxygen, destroyed by pasteurization and cooking, but preserved by steaming, somewhat affected by alkalies.	C —Pyorrhea (bleeding, sore gums), scurvy (wrinkles), easy bruising, hives, hay fever and skin infections, feelings of weakness, tender joints, inflamed and infected eyes and cataracts, shortness of breath, headache.	C —Sprouted seeds, young growing plants, apples, oranges, papayas, persimmons, fresh pineapple, rose hips, (green) Puerto Rican cherry juice, bean sprouts, broccoli (leaf), collards, kale, parsley, green peppers, guavas, lamb's quarters, cucumber, grapefruit, rhubarb, spinach, tomato, cabbage, asparagus, carrot, radish, strawberries, bananas.
D —(Other names of artificially produced D2 Vit. ergosterol, viosterol (calciferol), dehydrocholesterol) ENERGY, TOOTH & BONE FORMATION, NERVE-RELAXER. Insoluble in water, soluble in fats and oils, not affected by air or alkalies.	D —Buck and crowded teeth, knock knees, pigeon chest, rickets, "soft" bones, cramps and muscle twitching, fatigue, "nerves", near sightedness, arthritis, loss of calcium in the system.	D —Is the catalyst of calcium, so that the whole calcium family should be taken as well, if deficiencies exist: calcium, phosphorus, Vit. D and F, iodine, phosphatase. SUNLIGHT is the best source (do not shower for 5-6 hours after exposure), sunlamps in rainy weather, COD LIVER and other fish liver oils, egg yolks and milk (better in the summer).
E —(Alpha-tocopherol)-REPRODUCTION AND SUCCESSFUL PREGNANCIES, GLANDULAR HEALTH, HORMONE PRODUCTION, MUSCLE PERFORMANCE, ANTITOXIC, CARDIO-VASCULAR SYSTEM, GOOD FIGURE (pelvis & bust), PREVENTS THROMBOSIS IN LEGS. Insoluble in water, soluble in oils, not affected by light or heat, destroyed by chlorine.	E —Miscarriage, sterility, muscle degeneration and inflammation, lumbago, bursitis, rheumatism, heart attacks, has been helpful in phlebitis, gastric ulcers, muscular distrophy, multiple sclerosis, menstrual problems.	E —Fresh wheat germ oil, most vegetable oils, fresh cod-liver oils, sardines, shark-liver oil, barley, oatmeal, rye, yellow corn-meal, 100% whole wheat bread, brown rice, butter, eggs, cheese, fish, soybeans, navy beans, kale, parsley, yeast, sweet potatoes, brussels sprouts, leeks, carrots, turnip greens, spinach, watercress, celery, lettuce, apples, bananas, beef liver, kidneys, brain.

MINERALS

Without the proper mineral balance in our bodies we cannot survive. More attention is given to vitamins but many minerals are absolutely essential. I read with interest that doctors fortified the astronauts' diet with potassium to avoid minor heart problems. The following minerals are the most important.

BENEFITS	DEFICIENCY SYMPTOMS	FOOD SOURCES
CALCIUM: Is needed for Vit. D absorption, helps in blood-clotting, promotes regular function of heart muscle, nerve-relaxer, teeth and bone formation. Calcium is especially effective if the Vit. B complex, phosphorus, Vit. D, unsaturated fatty acids, iodine and phosphates are present in the diet.	Poor teeth, stunted growth, "nerves", muscle-spasms, convulsions, cramps, nail-biting, debility, rapid heartbeat, buck teeth, etc.	Milk, leafy greens such as beet greens, broccoli, Swiss chard, kale, collards, watercress, dandelion green, lettuce, spinach, blackberry, cabbage, carrot, celery, cranberry, figs, grapefruit, lemon, orange, rhubarb, parsley, turnip, mustard greens, beans, soybean flour, molasses, bone meal, almonds, cheese, barley-water.
CHLORINE: Is needed for hair growth, body-cleansing and by the digestive juices. It keeps joints flexible and helps in fat-reducing.	In animals: loss of hair, slow growth, apprehension and fear.	Raw meat, salt, milk, legumes, tomatoes, radishes, beets, ripe olives are all good sources.
COPPER: Is needed for the utilization of iron to prevent anemia.	Weakness and poor respiration.	Molasses, liver, oysters, clams, egg yolk, dried fruits (apricots), leafy vegetables, fresh fruit, soy flour, whole wheat grains and loganberries.
IRON: Is needed by every cell for oxygen supply; rosy complexion, vitality, resistance to infection. Chlorophyll is essential in the diet for adequate utilization of iron.	Anemia, fatigue, a gray, wrinkled face, dull hair, flat, cracked fingernails, a sore tongue and mouth and shortness of breath.	Uncooked leafy greens, liver, brewer's yeast, wheat germ, blackstrap molasses, peanuts, all fresh fruits, particularly apricots, soybeans, egg yolks, parsley, tongue, Swiss chard, clams, heart, kidneys, spinach, dates, whole wheat flour, beet greens, beans, bean sprouts, watercress, cabbage, tomatoes, turnips.

IODINE: Is needed for the smooth functioning of the thyroid gland which is the weight regulator of the body.	Sluggishness, overweight, goiter.	It is found in all seafoods such as cod, haddock, cod-liver oil, oysters, sardines, kelp, dulse, lettuce, potatoes, asparagus, cabbage, carrots, cranberry, cucumber, pineapple, prune, radish, spinach, tomato, watercress, apple, orange, sea salt on foods.
MAGNESIUM: Is especially needed for nerve-relaxation (in conjunction with calcium for depression), and muscle work. It strengthens bones and teeth, and has cholesterol dissolving properties, which in turn dissolve kidney and gallstones. It is also successfully used in treatment of coronary disease, polio, and epilepsy, and helps to prevent constipation, and upset tummy and poor circulation.		Nuts (almonds, cashews, peanuts), milk, egg yolk, whole wheat, legumes, lima beans, brown rice, spinach, dates, raisins, grapefruit and orange.
PHOSPHORUS: is the brother to Calcium and is needed to harden and strengthen bones and teeth, is in every cell but is especially prevalent in the brain and sex cells, keeps hair, nails and skin healthy, maintains the alkalinity of bloodstream, helps to form lecithin.	Poor teeth, poor appetite, weight loss, rickets, stunted growth, feeling of weakness.	Protein foods such as meats, milk, eggs, cheese, peas, nuts, soybeans, beans, legumes and all whole grains. For better utilization the diet should also be adequate in hydrochloric acid (B-vitamin complex, specifically thiamin), Vit. D, unsaturated fatty acid and phosphatose.
POTASSIUM: Is needed to balance the supply of food to and disposal of wastes from the cells.	Constipation, "nerves" in the form of insomnia, slow heartbeat, damaged heart muscles and kidneys, infant diarrhea, edema.	Most fruits and vegetables (potatoes) are good sources as are black molasses, almonds and figs, watermelon, bananas, prunes, olives, milk.
SODIUM: Is needed to control the acid-alkaline balance of the blood, keeps calcium in solution and aids potassium in its function.	Retarded and slow growth and underweight, heart-stroke, etc. Too much, however, causes hypertension and water-retention.	Muscle meats and most vegetables. It is better to derive it from natural sources and sea salt than table salt. Whole wheat grains, breads, cheese, buttermilk, spinach, watercress, celery, beets, lettuce and bananas are good sources.
SULPHUR: Is needed to promote the beauty of hair, skin and nails, it has a cleansing effect on the blood and affects body-resistance and liver absorption of minerals.		It is found in some proteins, milk, cheese, eggs, nuts, cabbage, Brussels sprouts, cereals and most fruits and vegetables.

INDEX